Beyond Boo-Boo Kisses: Beating Cancer at Death's Door

by
Leslie Graham

Published by Robby Graham Foundation, Largo, FL 33778

All Scripture quotations, unless otherwise indicated, are taken from the King James Version of the Bible (KJV).

Cover Design: Jeff Martens, Martens Creative
Front Cover Photography: Roni Puckett, Dream Makers Studios

Printed in the United States of America.

ISBN-10: 0615470408
ISBN-13: 978-0615470405 (Robby Graham Foundation)

DEDICATION

This book is dedicated to all who are hurting.
May you find a Comforter in its pages, Hope in its words,
and be embraced by the arms of Love

CONTENTS

FOREWORD

This is a beautiful book, because of its author's humility. This is a story of her 'son of G-d', her family of worship and her faith. As a young physician, my mentors taught me patience, so did my patients and their parents. Many holy men and women taught me prayer, so did my patients and their families.

I was taught the meanings of life by my rabbis and their 'Old Testament'. I kept learning the meanings of life by my patients, their families and their 'New Testament'. Old, New, Ongoing testament is Robby's story of recovery through worship.

Leslie Graham teaches us that no patient is ever alone, no family is ever abandoned. As I said to the Graham family fifteen years ago "Whatever you're doing, Keep doing it!"

Louis W. Solomon, MD
Assistant Professor Psychiatry
University of Florida
(Formerly, Robby's Pediatric
Neurosurgeon)

LESLIE GRAHAM

1
THAT WORD

That word alone strikes fear into all who receive its diagnosis. Immediately the questions come: Can it be cured? How long do I have? Is the prognosis certain? More questions than answers. Thankfully, I would be spared the pain, fear, and anguish of receiving such a diagnosis—for now.

"Well, the good news, Mrs. Graham . . . it's not cancer," the surgeon reported. Cancer? I didn't even know it was a possibility. What was happening? Only two weeks ago, I gave birth to a beautiful baby girl. In all my twenty-seven years, I had never had a major health challenge. Now I was lying in a hospital with tubes entering nearly every orifice.

"The bad news is . . . we don't know *what* you have. There's a mass in your gut that we can't identify, so I'd like to do additional tests, possibly exploratory surgery."

As a registered nurse, I processed this information. *Okay, not cancer. They're just going to check out some other things.* As the next days progressed, I thought I fully understood the complexities of the situation, not knowing that my husband was told I might not survive. My body was in immense pain, but my heart ached even more. Although my mother stayed with me 24-7, and my wonderful husband, Rick, visited me daily with our three beautiful children (once doctors determined I wasn't infectious), I longed to be home. I especially wanted to hold my new baby.

We finally had our little girl. She was the first girl born into the Graham family in over thirty years. With her strawberry blonde hair, blue eyes, and cute button nose, Amanda was the perfect mixture of both her brothers, and they loved her very much. Ricky, our oldest, was already seven years old. He had brown hair and blue eyes, the spitting image of his father. Robby favored my side of the family, his light blond, surfer-cut hair always bouncing as he tirelessly ran. He had blue eyes, instead of green like me, and the longest eyelashes you've ever seen. Why do boys always get the long eyelashes anyway?

Thanksgiving was quickly approaching and I had already spent Robby's birthday in the hospital. Four years old. How did time move so fast, and why couldn't I get well with that same speed?

Normally I wouldn't burden God with my petty needs. I knew the world was big and there were plenty of others whose needs far exceeded mine. In my profession, I often witnessed firsthand the pain, sickness, and death of this world. Certainly God had better things to do than be concerned about the many repairs our home needed or our empty bank account. I only bothered Him when I really needed something. This way, when I sent up a request, He knew I was serious. Generally, I lived my life and let Him live His. Now, however, I really needed Him. I couldn't get myself out of this one. In the hazy moments between morphine-induced periods of sleep, I wheeled and dealt with God, pleading for how good I would be if only He would let me live.

Stretching my arms toward the ceiling, I yawned as I rolled out of bed. My deadly encounter (and recovery) from six months earlier a distant memory, life was now permeated with bliss. Even the noisy alarm clock couldn't stop me from enjoying the day that lay ahead. As I cracked open the blinds, my eyes, barely open and still slightly crusted from sleep, were forced to realize the brilliance of the sun. I felt joy radiate from me as the sun and I exchanged beams. The beauty of the day confirmed that the universe was as thrilled as I.

I loved my job but cherished my days off even more. Being home with my family was the highlight of my week. Of course, working full time meant spending some of my weekend running errands. This particular day, when I returned from my errands, Rick was waiting.

"You can't believe what this kid did today," Rick said.

I looked up to see Robby playing happily in spite of the obvious scrapes and cuts to his face and lip. "What happened?"

"He kept standing up on the couch. Even after I yelled at him several times to get down and stop jumping on the furniture, he did it again. I turned away for a minute and then, for no reason at all, bam! He jumped face-first into the wall."

"Is he alright?" I asked. *This wouldn't have happened if I were home*, I thought. Rick was a cautious and protective father. In fact, sometimes he sheltered the kids too much. He'd never let anything bad happen to our children, but I couldn't stop feeling like I could've done better, had I been there. I scooped Robby up in my arms as he showed me his boo-boos.

"Here . . . let Mommy kiss it and make it all better," I said.

He tilted his cute little face up toward mine. Gently I kissed his scrapes. He smiled approvingly and ran off to play.

Rick continued his report. "He bloodied his nose and lip a little bit, that's all. At first I was worried that he had broken his nose. He hit the wall that hard. I asked him what the hell he was doing, but he was crying—"

"Awww, Rick, what did you yell at him for?" I interrupted.

"I don't know. Crazy kid. Well, I took him into the bathroom and cleaned him up. He was tired, so I put him in bed. He slept for a few hours."

"He slept for a few hours?" I was puzzled. Robby was always active and rarely took time to sleep. He had been that way since he was born. A very resilient child, at times he would fall, his body crashing to the ground. The sound alone hurt me more than the fall hurt him. He'd get up and keep on going, shaking it off like it was nothing. So it was strange to me that he would sleep at all, let alone for several hours.

"But he's alright now," Rick finished.

"Yeah, well, you owe the cup a quarter," I said, pointing at the cuss cup we had established. Cussing was getting out of hand for the two of us, and I thought it was a great way to save up for our vacation.

Later that day, I noticed that Robby's left eye appeared slightly crossed when he looked at me from a certain angle. I shrugged it off, thinking it was my imagination, but by Monday it was getting worse.

Tuesday afternoon was the earliest appointment we could get with the ophthalmologist. When I picked Robby up from preschool that afternoon, his eye had become noticeably crossed, now obvious to all who saw him.

"His optic nerves are inflamed and I'm not sure why," the ophthalmologist told us.

This was frustrating. He was a specialist. Why didn't he know what was going on?

He proceeded, "I'm going to send you over to Children's Hospital for a CT scan of his head. It's probably just an infection."

I rolled my eyes and sighed. "We have to go tonight?"

Rick, a fire captain, was still in uniform, and I had come straight from work as well. After nine hours in a suit, I was uncomfortable and tired. It had been a long day and I just wanted this over with.

The doctor continued, "I'm sure going there will probably ruin your plans for the evening, but it'll be worth it so we can all sleep well tonight."

I hated going downtown; it always felt gloomy and creepy. I certainly wasn't thrilled with the idea of sitting in the emergency room for any portion of the evening, but we had to know what the problem was. An uneasy feeling swirled in the pit of my stomach.

"I hate hospitals," Rick declared as we left the clinic.

"I know. And I hate going downtown too."

"I'm going home and changing into something more comfortable first."

"Not me. I'm leaving my suit on," I responded. "If there's one thing I've learned, it's that they'll treat you altogether different down there, depending on how you look. Otherwise, we'll end up getting treated like the rest of the flippin' indigents."

"You're right. I didn't think of that."

"Well," I sighed, glancing into my purse. "I picked the wrong day to quit smoking. I only have two cigarettes left."

"We're not stopping to buy more!" he snapped.

Quickly, we grabbed a bite to eat, and left Ricky and Amanda with Rick's mother before heading down to the hospital. Once there, we were placed in a small examination room in the emergency area. It had a gurney on one wall and just enough room for two chairs, one on each end of the gurney. Robby was given his own pint-sized patient gown. Wearing it didn't bother him a bit. He liked it because it was green.

For hours, doctors and nurses filed in to take their turns with Robby, who seemed unfazed. In fact, he took pleasure in being the center of attention. Everyone that entered our room enjoyed being entertained by this lovable kid who tried hard to make each of them laugh.

He was given an IV so they could administer medication, as well as the contrast medium for the scan. I couldn't believe how well he took it when she put it in. What a champ. He was certainly a better patient than I.

When it was time for his scan, Robby was given a dose of medicine for conscious sedation. Rick held him as the drug was pushed into his IV. Within moments, Robby became visibly tipsy, resembling someone who had too much to drink. As his body became limp, his eyes widened. Robby gazed up, pointing at his father and slurred, "Are you the mommy or the daddy?"

We all laughed, giving us a brief respite from the intensity of the evening's events.

Wrapped in lead vests, we stood next to Robby as he lay on the scanner table. Rick encouraged him to lie still while I repeatedly affirmed what a wonderful job he was doing. The sedative seemed to be working. I hadn't seen him lay that still since he was a baby.

As I looked down on him, my mind drifted off. I remembered him as a sleeping infant, so small and innocent. He was still my baby. It seemed only yesterday that I was changing *his* diapers. But staying a baby was definitely not Robby's plan. He was walking by the time he was eight months old, running by nine, and he hadn't stopped since. When he was a year old he started insisting, "Robby do it." Independent from the start, he radiated a joy and free-spiritedness that attracted you beyond his handsome looks.

Standing next to him at the scanner, we were able to see through a window into the room where the technician operated the equipment. At first she was in there alone. Then a person, who appeared to be a doctor, came in, then another person and another.

I began to worry the next time I glanced through the window. The room was now packed with doctors, all looking at the screen and shaking their heads. Fear began to invade my thoughts.

What is going on? Not one person would look toward us. My heart began to sink in my chest. I knew that this was not a good sign, but I was hoping for confirmation that my fears were imaginary.

"What are they doing in there?" I asked Rick.

"I don't know," he whispered as he glanced to the window, then returned to staring lovingly at Robby lying peacefully still on the table. "Are you doing alright, buddy?" Rick asked. Robby nodded his head yes.

Next, I saw Robby's nurse enter the technician room. I knew she would give it away; nurses always do. She looked first to the picture on the machine. Then she looked through the window toward us. She was the only one willing to look at us. The expression on her face made it easy to see the sorrow and pity she felt. Half of me was dying to know what they saw; the other half didn't ever want to know. I just wanted to go home. They'd told us the scan would only take about six minutes, but now we'd been in there twenty, which already seemed like an eternity. After they removed Robby from the scanner, they still were silent. We were sent back to our room to await the results.

Time crept and by 7:00 all three of us were ready to go home. The door to our room remained open and I kept looking out, hoping to see someone coming to relieve our anxiety and send us home. I had a gnawing pain in my stomach that I blamed on hunger, unwilling to acknowledge any other possibility.

Then I noticed a pleasant-looking, bearded gentleman strolling leisurely throughout the emergency unit. Eventually he came into our room, apparently looking for friendly conversation.

"Hi. I'm Dave, one of the hospital chaplains. Who is this handsome little guy?"
I should have known this visit was not by coincidence, but I had no clue what was really going on. I never suspected the chaplain was there for us. We chatted for a while and Dave spent some time amusing Robby. A child life specialist was still sitting on the gurney with Robby, entertaining him with her puppet. She had come in earlier to teach Robby about the IV put in for the scan, and she used the puppet to demonstrate. He was laughing and having a good time.

Finally the emergency room attending doctor was at our door. I stood to greet her.

"Mr. and Mrs. Graham, we're ready to give you a report," the doctor said. Her eyes revealed the regret of the impending news. "Are you ready?"

Hesitantly, I nodded my head yes as Rick stood up.

We left Robby and followed her, the initial doctor, and Dave to another room around the corner. My heart raced. I forced back the tears threatening to well up in my eyes.

The tiny four-by-eight room barely had space for two love seats in the corner. A counter and sink flanked the opposing wall, with the door where we entered completing the cramped quarters. There was barely room for standing.

I didn't like this tiny room. There were no windows, and the walls seemed to close in on us from every side. Rick sat down in one love seat, while I stood near him. The five of us packed in from wall to wall. No one else could fit—not even God.

The doctor closed the door. "Please, have a seat," she said.

I refused. "I'll stand," I answered, thinking that my standing would somehow change the words I was about to hear.

"Please—sit," the doctor repeated firmly.

Resolutely, I stood with my arms crossed, staring at her angrily. The doctor, her eyes fixed on mine, silently waited for my response. Her seemingly eternal pause finally urged me to be seated.

Reluctantly I eased myself down next to Rick. Sitting on the edge of the seat, my arms still crossed, I leaned forward, ready to listen.

2
THE WORST DAY EVER

The doctor inhaled deeply. "Mr. and Mrs. Graham," she paused, "your son has a brain tumor."

I gasped, trying to retrieve the oxygen that had just been knocked out of me. An unseen force squeezed my ribs, paralyzing my chest, while a pain like none I had ever felt ripped my heart into chunks. My hands found their way to my cheeks, tears streaming down my face. Time stood still. The tiny room seemed to close in further around us. My whole world became surreal. Pain flooded my body and my mind, blocking even a single thought.

I looked at Rick and he at me, both our eyes swelling with tears, neither of us knowing what to say. Nothing in life had prepared us for this. Our attention turned back to the doctor.

"Are you sure?" Rick asked.

"Yes, we are sure. There is definitely a tumor."

"Now what do we do?" I asked.

"We've already called Dr. Solomon," she answered. "He's the pediatric neurosurgeon. He'll be able to give you a more definitive prognosis."

We stared at her in silence. The uncomfortable pause urged her to continue. "For now, let's get you and Robby settled in a room. We'll give you a few minutes to talk and absorb everything."

I stood up, tears pouring over my cheeks. Oblivious to my surroundings, I somehow found a tissue and wiped away the tears. "I need a cigarette," I sobbed.

Chaplain Dave walked us to an area outside the back door and stayed to talk with us. He was especially encouraging and gave us reason to hope. After inhaling two cigarettes in quick fashion, I still needed more time to collect myself. I couldn't let Robby see me crying. I didn't want to scare him. I had to be strong.

I went back in and tried calling family. The only person I could reach was my friend Pat. We'd graduated from nursing school together, becoming good friends in the process. We even worked together until my recent job change. She decided to come to the hospital and stay with me while Rick went to tell his mother the bad news.

Rick and I returned to the room where Robby still waited. He was playing and hadn't missed us a bit. We explained that he would get to sleep over at the hospital for a few days. He thought that was neat.

"I'm just going to stay here for free days, Mommy," he said, holding three fingers in the air.

He could count to three, but he had no concept of what three days was going to be. I wished it would be only three days.

Robby was admitted to a private room and Rick left to tell his mom in person. Before long, Pat arrived to keep us company. I was so grateful I wouldn't have to stay alone. I was even more grateful when I saw a whole carton of cigarettes in her hands, just for me.

Around ten o'clock that night, Rick returned. The surgeon arrived soon after—a tall, thin man whose brown hair and mustache were streaked with bits of gray, revealing signs of age and experience. He wore a shirt and tie covered by a navy blazer, tan slacks, and his trademark cowboy boots. He strode into the room with a confidence bordering on arrogance.

"Hi folks! I'm Dr. Solomon," he announced as he walked into the room. Firmly he insisted, "First, let me tell you, your boy will be going home." He was friendly, factual, and had a strong air of assurance that floated throughout the room, landing on each of us. Showing us pictures from Robby's scan, he described the tumor and its position in terms we could understand, and then proceeded to assure us he would be able to get a good resection with minimal, if any, side effects. We discussed the three types of tumors he thought it could be.

The first possibility he mentioned was a slow-growing tumor called astrocytoma, which might not require any further treatment. The second type of tumor was called medulloblastoma, a much faster-growing tumor that would require chemotherapy and radiation. The third was the most malignant, and odds of survival were significantly decreased.

"More than likely, it's one of the first two," Dr. Solomon stated. "We are going to get Robby scheduled for surgery, because either way, it's got to come out."

By the time he left, we felt much better. Dr. Solomon had shined a little hope into our impossible situation. Surgery was scheduled for Thursday at noon, two days away.

Only one of us could sleep at the hospital with Robby. Wisely, he chose his daddy, who undoubtedly would keep him safe. When I got home, our house was disturbingly empty and quiet. Nothing seemed real—the events of the night still a blur. Lying in bed, I flipped through TV channels with the remote until falling asleep.

The sound of the morning news awoke me. Jolting upright in bed, I looked around the empty room. "It wasn't a dream," I said aloud to myself.

As I realized the magnitude of my new reality, rivers of tears began to soak my sheets. I had never cried so hard.

"Oh God," I cried, "help me!"

I lay in bed awhile, crying out my pain, until eventually I realized I had not yet told my family, and it was already past the time I usually left for work. I picked up the phone and dialed. One by one I called my family, Robby's school, and my employer. The reaction was always the same—the news was met with loud voices of disbelief, crying, gasping, and screaming. How do you ease the pain of others when your own pain is so alive?

I packed some things for Ricky and Amanda and then went to visit them for a few minutes. I drove to Rick's mom's on autopilot, having driven this route many times before. My mind was preoccupied with unlimited questions. *How will I explain this to Ricky?* He was only seven years old. And Amanda. *How can my six-month-old baby understand why Mommy and Daddy aren't around very much?* Surely the hospital would now consume our time. *Will Amanda miss Robby?* He would miss her. He loved playing with her and hugging and kissing her. *If he has chemo and radiation treatments, will he be able to touch her?* So many questions invaded my mind.

I arrived at the hospital to find Robby playing video games in his room. Soon he would be able to go to the playroom.

"I'm gonna stay here two more days, Mommy!" he said excitedly, holding up two fingers.

I tried to force a smile. "It might be a little longer, Rob."

How do you explain to a four-year-old that there is something deadly inside him, and the nice doctor is going to cut his head open and take it out so he'll feel better? He had no concept of what surgery was.

Rick was sitting on the side of the bed, clearly as distressed about everything as I was.

"How'd you sleep?" I asked.

"We didn't get much sleep," he answered.

I nodded, fully understanding why he might not have slept well.

"I laid in bed holding Robby all night. But the nurses were in and out of here a lot, and they put that apnea monitor on him to make sure he kept breathing." He bent over with his face in his hands. "This sucks!"

The doctor had told us the tumor in Robby's head was blocking the flow of cerebrospinal fluid. Robby should have been in serious pain, but he'd denied having a headache.

"How do you feel today?" I asked him.

"Fine, Mommy . . . let's go to the toy room," he said, bubbling with excitement.

There were many arrangements to be made prior to surgery, tons of papers to read and sign. While I took Robby to the toy room, Rick spent the morning on the phone, arranging for direct blood donors, just in case. Afterward, he left for the blood bank to sign the papers.

At 1:00, Robby and I went downstairs for his MRI. The doctors needed these pictures to get a better view of the tumor and to find out more about the configuration. Because their MRI unit was being revamped, we were escorted to a portable unit, housed in a trailer located right outside the emergency room.

"Sorry, you can't stay," the nurse informed me. "It'll only take about twenty minutes. Why don't you go walk around for a few minutes and we'll see you soon?"

I was afraid to leave him. I didn't want Robby out of my sight.

An hour and a half later, I saw the doors open on the side of the trailer. I was standing inside the emergency room, looking out through the glass doors. The attendants with Robby could not see me, but I could see them. As the door opened, I saw Robby cradled in the arms of one of them. She was transferring him to the stretcher while talking to her peer. I watched in horror as they dropped his head against the side rail. *Are these people stupid?* I raged to myself. It wasn't bad enough he had a tumor in his little head, but now they were shaking it up.

Did I say anything when they came through the doors? No. I had enough to deal with. Robby looked okay and I just couldn't bring myself to confront more trouble. We returned to the room, and the two attendants assured me they could handle watching him while I went to get the nurse. What could it hurt? He was still asleep from his sedation and he was already transferred into his bed. Surely they could be trusted to stand next to him and make sure he didn't fall out.

I found the nurse and told her we were back. Returning to Robby's room, I heard a loud bang followed by his screaming cry as I approached the door.

"What happened?" I shouted as I rushed in. If looks could kill, I would have never gotten an answer, because the two of them would have been lifeless on the floor.

"I don't know. He just sat up and slammed his head against the rail," the female attendant said.

At that moment, Robby's body flung up in bed. He screamed and threw himself down again. The monitors, still attached to him, beeped and shrieked all kinds of noises. I tried to calm Robby, but there was no reasoning with him. The nurse came in to see about all the commotion.

"What is wrong with him? Why is this happening?" I asked, fearing that thing in his head was already taking over his mind.

"The medication they use for sedation in the MRI can sometimes cause temporary psychosis in children," the nurse explained.

"Are you serious?! Why would they use it then?"

Robby continued to scream and throw himself around intermittently. I picked him up from the bed and rocked him in the rocking chair. He would fall asleep for a while, then suddenly wake up and start screaming again. I held him tightly as over and over he would kick and scream, his limbs flailing in every direction like he was possessed. Hours passed. My arms grew weaker. I didn't know if I could continue holding on.

Please, God, help me, I begged silently. *Please make him stop. Make this go away. I'll do whatever you want me to do, just fix my little boy!* I rocked and I pleaded. This wasn't fair! It was enough having to deal with my baby boy getting diagnosed with a horrible disease. While I was still recovering from that announcement, I had to deal with him being in a state of psychosis. *Where is Rick? Why is it taking him so long? How much longer do I have to do this?*

I rocked and rocked. Robby would sleep awhile, but then he'd wake up and scream and hit and kick. Occasionally he'd rest and cry, but then the screaming and kicking would start again. Over and over the cycle repeated—for hours. His nurse stayed in the room almost the entire time. She would leave only long enough to check on her other patients.

All this time, Robby's vital signs were unstable. They would shoot way above normal when he was awake screaming, then drop dangerously low when he fell asleep. Four hours later, the nurse had Robby transferred to the intensive care unit. She was uncomfortable caring for him any longer due to his vulnerable condition. Rick returned just as the decision was made to move him.

"What took you so long?" I demanded.

"I went as fast as I could. It just took a long time to get everything taken care of."

I knew he was trying to do his best, but I was tired and angry, already worn down from the stress of the situation. He took over rocking Robby so I could rest. Fortunately for Rick, the screaming and kicking seemed to vanish, reduced to an occasional whimper. Moments later, Robby was transferred to the ICU. He would receive individualized attention there at least, and the nurses were more qualified to care for his condition. We made sure he was safely tucked in, and then as Robby quietly slept, we decided to go and talk to Chaplain Dave.

Surgery was less than a day away, and we wanted to ask Dave to baptize Robby before surgery. We were members of a Catholic church, but it never occurred to us to call them. We were so numb from the preceding twenty-four hours that I'm surprised we even thought of baptism.

Dave happily invited us into his office and asked us for an update. This was good because it gave us time to think of a way to ask about the potential baptism. Just as Rick began to speak, a Catholic priest knocked on Dave's open door.

"Could you help me?" he asked Dave. "I'm looking for Mr. and Mrs. Richard Graham."

Dave turned and looked at the two of us and then, smiling, looked back to the priest. "This is Mr. and Mrs. Graham right here."

"I'm here to baptize your little boy. Are the godparents present?"

Rick and I looked at each other, stunned and speechless. How did he know? It was really strange. I looked around to see if someone was watching.

"Uh . . . my sister's here," I stammered, "but nobody else."

"That's okay. We'll find a Catholic nurse or someone to be a stand-in."

Like two zombies we got up and silently followed the priest to Robby's bedside. As we walked down the hall, Rick looked at me, his big blue eyes questioning me. I shrugged my shoulders and whispered, "My mom must have called."

Was it divine intervention or amazingly coincidental timing? I didn't know. At any rate, Robby was christened at his bedside in the intensive care unit of the hospital. Quickly, and without emotion, the priest completed the baptism. Robby slept through the entire short-lived ceremony.

Afterward, we forced ourselves to eat something at the cafeteria. We returned from dinner to find Robby sitting up, smiling, and eating his own dinner. Dr. Solomon was at his bedside. As we discussed the MRI results, I proceeded to ask a zillion questions. The nurse in me was coming to life! He answered to the best of his ability, but there was still so much unknown.

He told me we need not change our vacation plans for July. "He should be perfectly able to go on a vacation by that time. Don't change anything. Let's just take it one day at a time right now," he said.

Dr. Solomon was incredibly reassuring and confident. Somehow that eased my fears, but it didn't take them away.

Because Robby was stable, Dr. Solomon had him transferred back to his room upstairs. I stayed until midnight and then returned to my empty home once again.

The house was a disaster. I was tired, but I couldn't resist cleaning up a bit. Some of Robby's toys were lying on the family room floor. I opened the door to his room to put them away. We'd recently finished remodeling, and both boys were excited about sleeping in their new bunk beds.

Their dinosaur-themed room reminded me of the joy the boys had playing with each other. They were the best of friends. I lay on the bottom bunk snuggled up to Robby's now tear-stained pillow. *Will Robby ever sleep in his bed again?* I wondered. What would Ricky do without his little buddy? They did everything together.

3
IMAGINATION

Imagine the feel of your body, intruded by the cold, hard tip of a scalpel blade. Yes, you're fortunate enough to sleep through the invasion, but that doesn't stop the assault on your mind in the moments preceding surgery.

My mind reeled with images from my own surgery only six months earlier. Lulled into a quasi-zombie state, a combined effect of shock and exhaustion, my brain gave way to thoughts and images best left unspoken.

Envision a saw briskly intruding through your skull, the cracking of bone combined with the sucking sound of tissue releasing as the surgeon pops it back to reveal your brain sleeping peacefully inside.

I tried to block the images from my mind. Was this really happening?

Thursday arrived and still nothing seemed real. My baby boy was having brain surgery today.

The Ronald McDonald House would be our temporary home while Robby was in intensive care following surgery. Ricky and Amanda would remain with Rick's mother, whom they fondly called Nanu. That morning I made all of the necessary arrangements for our housing and then returned to the hospital to find Robby awake—and mad. He'd been given steroids to reduce inflammation, and an unfortunate side effect was an increased appetite. He was hungry and didn't understand or care that he was having surgery. He just wanted to eat!

After only two days in the hospital, Robby had changed dramatically. His eye was now severely crossed, causing him to turn his head sideways in order to see. His sweet face now resembled a cartoon character, and I felt my insides distress as I watched him. His balance was increasingly off and he frequently walked into things. It was most noticeable when he walked the straight empty hallway, his entire frame slanted to one side. I convinced myself this was due to his eyesight, completely denying the reality of his diagnosis. The child life therapist returned with her puppets to explain to Robby that he was going to have surgery that day. Yet it was impossible for him to truly understand what was about to happen.

Rick and I forced ourselves through the motions that morning. There was so much to do and no time to talk about how we felt. We concentrated on taking care of business; it kept our mind off our feelings. Moreover, I don't think we even knew how we felt. There was no spare time to think about that. We were focused on Robby. Our feelings would have to wait.

The operating room was behind schedule, adding to our stress level. I took Robby to the playroom to distract him from his hunger and distract myself from the impending pain. He tried to play, but things, which only yesterday he could do with ease, were now too difficult. Instead of distracting him, the playroom simply served to frustrate him further. We returned to his room, and finally transport came to escort him to the surgical holding area. My mother, Robby's Mema, arrived only seconds before.

In the hall outside Robby's room, we stood waiting for Rick to bring him out to the gurney.

"I want to talk to Robby for a minute," Rick said.

"Sure," the orderly answered.

I walked toward the room as Rick began closing the door. He nearly had it closed all the way when I pushed on it to let myself in. He held the door firmly, his eyes staring desperately into mine, his head shaking no.

"I want to talk to him alone," he urged.

I reluctantly nodded yes, hung my head, and stepped back from the door.

Several minutes later the two immerged, Rick's eyes red and watery. He tenderly placed Robby aboard the gurney while holding his own tears at bay.

Our arrival at the surgical holding area ended a solemn, quiet walk. Mema gave Robby hugs and kisses at the door and reminded him of the picnic they were going to have at the park when he got home.

Inside were three or four gurneys along the wall and a few rocking chairs on the opposite side. We quietly rocked in the chairs as the world hustled around us. Doctors, nurses, parents, and children constantly moved in and out. Robby snuggled on Rick's lap with his head laid back on his father's chest. Each of us consumed in our own thoughts, we barely spoke.

I watched several sets of parents and children revolve in and out the doors. One mom was upset to tears that her little girl was having tubes placed surgically in her ears. I jealously wished I could trade places with her.

One by one the anesthesiologist, nurses, physician's assistant—all those who would be participating in the surgery—came out to tell us how they would play their part. Finally Dr. Solomon came in, still carrying his overflowing confidence. Like a general about to enter war, he had total command of everything, including the nurses and other staff. Smiling, he approached us. "Your little boy will go home again. He's going to be just fine."

I wanted to believe him but knew the odds were stacked against us.

From Rick's lap, Robby gave each of us a hug and a kiss. We both struggled to hold back the tears. The priceless look of innocence on Robby's face pulled at my heart as his tiny hand stretched out to caress his father's face. He smiled softly and confidently reassured, "Don't worry Daddy, I'll be all right."

I watched helplessly as he and Dr. Solomon turned and walked hand in hand through the double doors to surgery. In awkward silence, Rick and I slowly made our way to the family waiting area.

The waiting area was loud and active, not the place for quiet solitude. Most of the seats were filled with anxious parents and grandparents, all waiting for their child to come out of surgery. We checked in with the receptionist and sat down. There weren't many words exchanged between my husband and I. Rick refused to leave the waiting area, in case someone came out. I couldn't sit still. I walked around the hospital or outside in the garden area. I'd get a soda from the cafeteria, make a quick stop now and again to the chapel, and then head back to the waiting area each hour for an update from the surgical nurse.

As I circled my way around the hospital once again, numerous thoughts invaded my mind, which seemed unable to keep pace with my rapidly changing emotions. At any given moment I was worried, scared, hopeful, frustrated. I tried to have a good, positive attitude. Something deep within made me feel like everything would, somehow, be all right. I didn't know how. I didn't even know why I felt that way. It didn't make any sense.

A program I'd watched the night before replayed in my mind. A nun, teaching about the many ways God shows us He is with us, described a budding flower as a symbol of life. It was one way, she said, that God displayed His promise to be with us, to make life new every day. I needed a flower bud.

As I walked I talked to God a lot, or should I say *at* Him? I asked plenty of questions without listening for answers, telling Him all of my frustrations and fears. He was an excellent listener, and it was a good thing He was there—I couldn't talk to Rick.

I didn't know what was going through my husband's mind, but he was anything but company. He sat slumped in the same chair all day. His eyes, bright red from lack of sleep, stared into the distance. His mind seemed to review the many thoughts that bombarded him also. On one of my stops in the waiting room, I reached out my hand to hold his and told him that it was going to be okay. He gave me a look of disbelief, and then his face dropped into his hands as he deeply sighed. The only one he really talked to was his mother, whom he called regularly to give updates. My mom must have felt very out of place. Rick wouldn't talk and I kept leaving.

The hours dragged by. I was exhausted, yet wired with nervous energy. For two days, I had barely slept or eaten. Caffeine and nicotine were my new best friends.

The first three hourly reports on Robby were uneventful. The fourth hour, the nurse came out, sat in a chair near Rick, and asked me to have a seat. I hate when they do that.

The initial pathology report had come back. The tumor was malignant and now *it* had a name—medulloblastoma. It was the second possibility we had learned of in those first hours. My heart became heavy in my chest. I leaned forward and held my face in my hands as I sighed.

My mother's eyes watered as she gasped, "No!"

Rick shook his head with anger and disbelief.

I'd truly believed it would be the first option, the one that required the least amount of intervention, maybe even something benign. How could this happen? I thought everything was going to work out. I was angry and hurt. Yet even while my heart ached, I still felt like Robby was going to be okay.

After the nurse left, we all sat in silence for a few minutes collecting our thoughts. Again I looked at Rick. "I still think he's going to be okay, honey," I said.

He lifted his head from his hands to look at me. "Would you quit saying that?" he replied angrily. "It's *not* okay!"

I couldn't comfort him. He had put his trust in the doctor, and that's who he wanted to tell him that everything was okay. Crying, I went back outside to the garden, talking to God as I went, a strong urge to fight rising within me.

I won't let this bring me down! I don't care what You allow me to come up against! The words screamed from my heart as my lips stayed silent. *I'm not ready to give up that easily. You're supposed to be a God of miracles!*

My God loved me and wouldn't let me down. With my God, *all* things were possible. That's what I'd been taught and I believed it. The problem was, I didn't know much else about my God. I didn't know His laws. I didn't read His Word. Until now, I didn't even have time for Him.

I spent the next hour on the garden patio talking with God during my chain-smoking session. Eventually my insistence—demanding He help me—changed to an attitude of submission.

Lord, I know Robby is Your child, and his fate is ultimately in Your hands. I can run around down here doing whatever I can, but without Your help, my efforts are pointless. I pleaded with God, *Please don't take my son. If I had my way, he would be healthy and we wouldn't be going through this right now, but I believe You know what is best for all of us.*

The story of Abraham and Isaac came to mind. My limited hours in Sunday school had seemingly begun to serve a purpose. I imagined what it must have been like for Abraham to offer up his one and only son, for whom he waited so long. Hesitantly I gave control of my son over to God too. At least I thought I did.

Lord, I pray you will heal him and make him well and he will have a long, healthy, normal life here on earth. No matter what Your decision is, I know You will give me what I need to deal with it.

It should have been easy. After all, I had just handed my son over to a man whose hands were right now inside of my child's brain. Who better to give Robby to than the One who knew every cell in his body?

Over eight hours had passed before Robby emerged from surgery. "Robby is doing fine," the nurse said. "The surgical team is moving him to ICU, and Dr. Solomon will be out in a little while to give you an update."

My sister Candy and her husband, Erik, had arrived, as well as my mom, my sister-in-law, Christine, and some family friends. About half an hour later, Dr. Solomon came in the waiting room. The stern look on his face made my heart race.

He formally began his report of the surgery. "We got about 90 to 95 percent of the tumor out. There were several small areas I could see growing into the vermis [the area between the cerebellum's two hemispheres]." He continued, "I could have removed more, but I may have been removing his ability to speak, and I think we can get it through chemo and radiation."

He told us the tumor itself was lying deep within the brain along the brain stem. "It didn't appear to be growing into the brain stem, but it was growing on it. I removed as much as I could and cauterized along the stem itself."

"Is he okay?" I asked.

"Robby did well during surgery, and we didn't have to give him any blood. Right now he is resting in ICU. He is responding somewhat, but is still coming out of sedation."

"Is he awake enough to talk to us?" Rick asked.

Dr. Solomon shook his head. "He's still coming out of the anesthesia. I've also ordered morphine and Valium to keep him from being in pain." He continued, "I want to tell you about how he looks so you won't be alarmed when you see him. He has a restraint on his right arm to keep him from pulling out any of the tubes and a catheter coming out of his head to drain the cerebrospinal fluid. Right now it has a blood-tinged color, but that's normal from the surgery. It should start to clear up over the next couple of days."

Rick and I listened intently as Dr. Solomon went on, "After a few days, we will see how he is doing and start taking steps toward removing the drain. He also has several IV lines and a urinary catheter. His face is very puffy and swollen from lying with his head down for several hours during the surgery, but that should start to subside over the next day or so, and it's actually not as bad as I would have expected."

I thought he would never stop.

"He also has a large bandage on the back of his head and neck, where we entered the head for the surgery. You'll probably notice he keeps his head to one side for the next few days to avoid pain. Don't worry, it's normal. Most of my kids do that." He paused and looked at us expectantly. "Do you have any other questions?"

In a daze, Rick and I shook our heads no.

"I've ordered consults with the oncology team. They will probably be coming to see you in a couple of days. The nurses are settling him in and they will come to get you when you can see him." He shook ours hands, saying, "I'll see you tomorrow."

That was it. Robby had survived the surgery. I was eager to see him, to know that he was okay. At the same time, I was afraid to see him, not really knowing what kind of condition he was in. When he went into surgery, he was walking and smiling. What would he be like now?

Finally the nurse came for us, informing us of the rules for visitors in ICU. Most of the intensive care unit was open. We looked into each bed as we walked past, trying to find Robby, wondering if we would recognize him. Then, at the end of the row of beds, the nurse entered a door to a private suite. Robby was inside.

My heart raced as we entered the room. There were tubes everywhere, machines intermittently beeping on and off. At the side of his bed was another nurse, vigorously writing notes. Robby lay motionless on his back. His face was red and puffy, his eyes almost swollen shut. He looked like he had just gotten out of a boxing match. The nurse directed us to the sink to wash our hands. Robby began to moan in pain. He tried to cry, hesitating as though it were too painful even to shed tears. Rick and I reached over to hold his hand.

"Robby . . . Mommy and Daddy are here, pumpkin," Rick whispered lovingly.

Robby whimpered and a tear rolled down the left side of his face.

Rick asked, "What's the matter? Are you hurting somewhere?"

"I just gave him some morphine," said the nurse.

He leaned over to Robby, "It'll be okay, pumpkin. The nurse will keep giving you medicine so you'll feel better. Okay?"

Robby was slow to answer. He seemed to be fading in and out of consciousness. On the outside, we were pillars of strength. On the inside, we were crumbling apart. Robby said only a few words to us that night. On occasion, he would move his leg or squeeze our hand. Then we noticed he wasn't moving his left side. I mentioned this to the nurse.

"I know. He hasn't moved that side since he's been out of surgery." She shrugged, "It happens sometimes."

I didn't like it, not one bit. But what did I know about brain surgery patients? Maybe it was a normal side effect. He would probably come out of it in a couple of days. From what I remembered of the potential side effects, many things were possible, but it was hard to tell which ones would be permanent until a few days after surgery. I felt trapped, at the mercy of the entire hospital. I was in no position to argue.

I'll see what the doctor says about it tomorrow, I thought.

We stayed with our son into the wee hours of the morning, waiting and hoping he would wake long enough to make us feel comfortable leaving him. Finally the nurse suggested we go to the Ronald McDonald House to get some sleep.

"He'll need you to be rested up for him tomorrow, and he'll probably sleep all night anyhow," she said. "He's the only patient I have, so I won't be leaving his side. I'll be sure he gets his pain medication every two hours."

"You go over. I'll stay here," Rick told me.

"You should go too," the nurse suggested. "You really need to rest."

Rick could barely keep his bloodshot eyes open, but he did not want to leave Robby for a moment. He had to make sure that he was taken care of.

"If he wakes up and asks for you, I'll call you right away. And besides, you're only a minute from us, right out the back door," she assured.

Rick looked out the window. Realizing how close our room was to the ICU, he was convinced to try and get a couple of hours of sleep.

We each took our turn kissing Robby and saying good-night. Gently holding his hand, my eyes rested on my baby boy. I wanted to hold him tight and take it all away, but Mommy's kisses couldn't heal this boo-boo.

4

WAR

The large green field, once blessed with the sweet smell of fresh pine from bordering forests, was now littered with piles of bodies. Blue uniforms to the north and grey to the south, a river of crimson formed a new union. The air was heavy with the residue of gunpowder as the smell of death permeated the atmosphere. Young men and old, the grim reaper held no bias. From dark corners men cried out, unable to help themselves, their limbs shredded, their insides hanging out. The sound of gunfire in the distance proved that someone somewhere continued the fight. What force can drive brother to kill brother? Father to kill son? Why? Why do men go to war?

Opposing forces rise, each believing they are right. When someone is passionate about change, enough to kill for the cause, enough to die for it, then war is imminent. The depths of my own passion were about to be tested, the battle lines soon to be drawn.

Early the next morning, I entered the ICU to find Rick talking to a tall, mature, African American gentleman. He reached out and shook my hand.

"Hello. I'm Dr. Cotman, the radiation oncologist. I wanted to stop in to introduce myself and talk to you about radiation therapy," he said.

27

"What are you doing here?" I asked suspiciously. I couldn't believe it. I wasn't ready to talk to an oncologist. Couldn't they let us recover for a few days? I didn't want to talk about *any* treatment, let alone radiation.

"I was asked to consult on your son's case," he replied.

"Who said he has to have radiation? I thought that this could be treated with chemotherapy?" I quizzed.

"Usually," he said calmly, "we treat these cases with a combination of chemotherapy and radiation. He can be treated with chemotherapy alone, but we find that it is much more effective to use the combination of therapies."

"Well, I'm not interested in talking about radiation right now," I said dismissively.

"I'll come back in a few days then."

"What is up with that?" I asked Rick after the doctor left.

"I don't know," he said, "he got here just before you did."

"How's Robby doin'?" I asked.

He shrugged his shoulders and looked down at Robby, who appeared to be sleeping. "I don't know. He's not talking today."

He reached over, delicately stroking Robby's arm. "Robby, Mommy's here," Rick said softly.

Robby shook his head, acknowledging my presence, still not opening his eyes.

Moments later another doctor came in.

"Hi. My name is Dr. Grana, I'm one of the oncologists here," she introduced herself with a European accent.

Are these flippin' people ever going to stop coming?

She spent a lot of time with us, trying to answer our countless questions. We desperately needed to know Robby's chances of surviving this ordeal.

"We expect standard risk candidates to have a 60–80 percent chance of survival."

"What constitutes standard risk?" I questioned.

"We consider a patient to be standard risk when there is only one tumor, no evidence of spread, and with a good resection of the tumor," Dr. Grana explained.

"So when will we know all that?" Rick asked.

"Robby will have an MRI of his head and spine. Then we will check his bone marrow and his skeletal x-rays, and perform some other tests," she answered.

"When are you going to do all of this?" I asked.

"Over the next few days . . . then we'll decide the best course of treatment for Robby, based on the results."

The best course of treatment? I thought to myself. *Oh, Lord.* I knew that life as I'd known it had forever changed. I couldn't go back, but I wasn't ready to cross over into this new world either. Riding the border between denial and reality, I reluctantly entered the discussion about treatment.

"What types of treatment?" I asked her.

"The standard treatment protocol at this time calls for a combination of chemotherapy drugs along with radiation."

Looking at her, I think she could tell I was less than thrilled with her answer.

"I'll be back again later to answer any more questions that you might have," she said.

Robby had not yet opened his eyes and wasn't moving his left side either. As the swelling began to dissipate, it became increasingly obvious that the entire left side of his face was flaccid. When he cried, only the right side of his mouth and face moved. My insides ached and I felt queasy as it became obvious that his left side was paralyzed. No one knew why or if it would ever change.

That afternoon, the assault continued with a visit by an oncology nurse. I walked with her to the family waiting area, the only place nearby to talk alone. I proceeded to ask her dozens of questions about treatments, side effects, and the like.

"What do you do as far as diet?" I asked.

"We believe that a well-balanced diet is all that these kids need," she replied.

So far I wasn't impressed by their servings of a "well-balanced diet." An average meal at this hospital consisted of processed chicken nuggets, macaroni and cheese, a mushy cooked vegetable, maybe a fruit, and always a sugary dessert.

"You mean to tell me that you don't give these kids any special kind of diet?"

She looked at me, puzzled, and responded, "Well, no. Why would they require a special diet?"

"So you beat these kids' immune systems up with chemo and radiation, and you don't do anything to help strengthen them?" I drilled.

"Like I said, we feel that a well-balanced diet is all they need. Most of these kids don't want to eat anything at all, so we're just happy to see them eating."

I was appalled. Cardiac patients get special diets to lower their risks; diabetics get special diets, as do a multitude of patients with other diseases. Why wouldn't they promote a healthier diet for cancer patients? They didn't even believe in giving multivitamins! Realizing that I wasn't going to get the answers I wanted, I politely dismissed her.

For one hour every evening, the ICU nurses changed shifts. During that hour, parents were required to leave. Back at the Ronald McDonald house that evening, Rick and I tried to pass the time. Our tiny room had two single beds, a small bathroom, and no television or radio. We were required to do a daily chore as a condition of our stay. I'm sure that it served to keep the house in order, and gave the parents something constructive to keep their minds off of their troubles—but we were *not* interested. I was fuming. How dare they ask me to clean up after other people when my own home sat in disarray? I was more interested in lying in a cave by myself.

The truth is, I didn't know how much time I had left with my son, and I didn't want to spend any time on someone else. All I could think about was my baby in the room across the street, and my two little ones at home whom I missed deeply.

Haphazardly, we completed our chore. Our hearts definitely weren't in it; we did it because we needed a place to stay.

Back in our room, I sat on one bed, reading through the literature the oncology nurse had given me. It was loaded with details about brain tumors, chemotherapy, and radiation therapy. My outward display of disgust cleverly veiled an inward fear that increased with each paragraph I read.

Rick lay on the opposite bed with his eyes closed, trying to rest.

"Hmm . . . side effects of radiation . . . hair loss, diarrhea, infertility, secondary cancer. Oh goodie, let's just kill cancer with a treatment that causes cancer. Sign me up! Can you believe this crap?" I ranted. "I can't believe they want me to do this to my son . . . and they don't even have a supportive diet."

Spans of total silence were interrupted with expressions of my disgust for our sole choice in therapy. Rick, in turn, would say he didn't want to talk about it. This went on for half an hour, when, dismissively, I flung the pages down on the bed. I couldn't read any more of that stuff.

My attention moved to the box of cards and letters that had begun to stream into the hospital, wishing Robby well. These would be nicer to read.

Rick sat up in his bed. "I can't sleep," he said. Rising to his feet, he stretched and sighed, "What are we going to do?" He paused. "How are we going to get through this?"

I stood and leaned in gently to hug him. His arms wrapped around me and held on so tight that I could barely breathe.

"I just can't stand the thought of losing him," he began to cry.

"We aren't going to lose him," I replied, trying to sound more sure than I actually was.

He released his grip, stood back a step, firmly grasping my upper arms.

"Why do you keep saying that?" he asked, somewhat irritated.

I stared intently into his watery eyes and answered, "I don't know how to explain it. I just have this feeling, deep down inside, that no matter how bad things look right now; it's all going to work out. We just have to have faith."

He began to cry, squeezing me tighter and tighter. "I wish I could have that much faith. I don't know how you do it, but I wish that I could just believe that he's going to be all right," he sobbed.

"You will," I said, unsure whether I believed it myself, "you will."

Days passed in the ICU, and things continuously got worse, each battle larger than the last. Monday came, with no changes in Robby's abilities. Results of his postoperative MRI indicated spread of disease to the spine—another blow to our hope. So far, nothing had gone our way.

How could it have spread to his spine so quickly? God, where are You? I prayed. *Maybe I am crazy,* I thought. *Maybe he's not going to get better. Perhaps I should start preparing for the worst.*

That afternoon, I went out to the garden to have a cigarette. The nominal stretch of space had become my personal sanctuary. It wasn't much to look at, its name deceptively masking the plainness of it all. Two round tables with benches sat on a dreary little slab of concrete which connected to a short sidewalk that wound briefly along the side of the building. Patches of greenery covered the surrounding ground and rose above the fence of the small area, the air always thick with clouds of secondhand smoke.

There were more people outside than usual, so I walked under the overhang to stand. Above me were the rooms of the second, third, and fourth floors. I paced back and forth, my mind engrossed by the latest bad report.

Thoughts attacked, none of which I should have been listening to. Then, from somewhere inside me, I heard, *"Look there."* I looked closely. Down, near the sidewalk, stood a tiny budding peace lily. My heart began to race. I had been looking for this sign for days! Fearing that this was just one of many flowers—and not a special sign God left only for me—I began combing through every part of the garden area. I found no other flowers anywhere, so I returned and stared at that precious little plant, my own message from heaven. Earlier I'd felt like giving up, my heart and soul wearing thin, then God sent me this assurance that He had not left me to fight alone. I rushed back in to share my news with Rick.

While I was out, things had taken an upward turn. The doctors had decided to move Robby to a regular room upstairs. He was still paralyzed on his left side, hadn't eaten or drank anything since the night before surgery, and was still not talking. But at least he was stable, they reasoned, and he'd spent four days in ICU, much longer than anticipated.

Soon after the move, however, Robby started having trouble breathing. They hooked him up to an apnea monitor, which would alarm if he quit breathing. Was this his asthma or another side effect? He hadn't moved in days; hopefully pneumonia wasn't setting in. Only one of us could stay with him now that he had his own room. Rick insisted it be him.

I returned to the hospital the next day to find that Robby's room had been changed again, to a private one. He cried frequently out of frustration to communicate. The nurse took out his catheter, deciding he needed to wear a diaper since he couldn't tell anyone he needed to go to the restroom. How humiliating for him. He didn't want to be treated like a baby.

That afternoon I took a walk down to the garden to visit "Robby's flower," as I began affectionately referring to it. It was still there, growing larger and healthier. To most it wouldn't have seemed like much, but to me it was a huge source of peace and assurance. As I sat on the bench, I looked up to the overhang above and realized that Robby's room was now directly above that little flower. I delighted in the fact that God had chosen that very spot and I hoped as the flower grew and strengthened, so would Robby.

However, with each passing day, it was our frustration that grew instead. Every day there was at least one new problem. The doctors gave us conflicting answers, sometimes even contradicting themselves. Interns changed orders, which Dr. Solomon then had to correct on his nightly rounds. Nurses seemed to have forgotten their training. They knew we watched everything they did, yet they continued to make mistakes.

Robby was still on an apnea monitor for fear he'd stop breathing. He was unable to swallow his own saliva, requiring us to suction his mouth frequently to keep him from catching pneumonia. Days passed, and still nothing was done to nourish him. He had IV fluids to keep him hydrated, but what were they going to do to get him eating? Rick refused to leave the hospital. He wouldn't budge from the room, even when I was there. He insisted on protecting Robby from any further problems. The nurses surely would've liked both of us to leave on occasion. We were constantly reminding them how to do their job.

The odds of Robby's survival continued to decline, compounding our disappointment. We didn't understand. What were the doctors basing their information on? Robby's tests continued to yield good results, yet each day the oncologists predicted a lower chance of survival. Hopelessness was winning.

Outside the hospital, all of creation continued on like nothing had ever happened. My life was falling apart while others lived on without a care, not even noticing that the world had forever changed. The sun, that everyone else was undoubtedly enjoying, annoyed me immensely. It was ever shining brightly, and I resented it for doing so. Didn't it know that everything was supposed to be much darker now?

Friends and family visited the hospital daily. Although they tried to bring us comfort, the right thing to say escaped them on many occasions. One day, an older, white-haired lady from my mother's church stopped in to encourage and pray for us. We sure needed it. She was nicely dressed and her pleasant personality brought a refreshing change. Being a cancer survivor herself, she oozed helpful information. I truly enjoyed her visit. I needed someone to believe with me. No one else seemed able.

On her way out, the woman leaned over to give me a hug and whispered in my ear, "Keep praying, honey, but remember, sometimes the answer is no."

In an instant I went from loving this lady to despising her. I was stunned. Here I was telling her how I believed that God was going to make everything right—how I just knew deep in my spirit that everything would work out—and then she betrayed me. Her words cut deeply like a knife in my heart and echoed in my mind, ". . . *sometimes the answer is no.*"

"That's what I've been telling you," Rick said when I complained about her negative remark.

I refused to believe it. Was her information wrong? It was for me. The whole world seemed to be against us. We were lone soldiers in need of allies. Could this war possibly be won? One thing was certain we loved Robby enough to fight the unknown battles that lay ahead, enough to kill for the cause, and enough to die for it. The war had begun.

5

THE ENCOUNTER

Wonderful things happen to each of us every day. The sun rising in the morning, butterflies erupting from cocoons, or a rainbow in the sky of a storm-ravaged city—these are but a few of the ordinary miracles that meet us on a daily basis. Yes, we all have encounters where people and events impact us. Sometimes they come from deep within, like the warmth that covers us as we hug a loved one, or the passion that pounds from our hearts during a favorite film while we silently observe the perfect couple united in love's first kiss. Other times we're impacted by forces outside ourselves, like when a mother sees a twenty blow by on the ground just as she's praying for her hungry children to be fed. Now and again, the most excellent things come unexpectedly, in the midst of hopelessness, when we're blessed with an encounter so glorious that life is forever changed.

A week after surgery, we were invited to conference regarding Robby's treatment plan. In light of the regular conflicts among the doctors, and the almost daily drop in our son's predicted survival rate, we were excited about the opportunity to speak to all of them together, at one time. We needed to hear their collective vision for conquering this enemy.

Rick left Robby to attend the conference only because a nurse he trusted promised to stay in the room with Robby until we returned. We opened the door to the conference room and stood in disbelief as shock and disappointment overcame us. Dr. Grana was the only one there.

"It is difficult to find a time for all doctors to be available," she explained in her thick European accent.

With reluctance we sat down with her. She reviewed all of the test results and the typical treatment options—a repeat of all we'd heard from them before.

"But he hasn't eaten for over a week and he looks so bad," Rick argued.

"I don't see how he can live through that kind of treatment," I rebutted. "We want him to have a quality life, as much as possible, for whatever amount of time he has left."

"Surgery, radiation, and chemotherapy are the standard protocols used for treatment," she repeated.

Our faces revealed frustration. Slouched back in our chairs, we were once again discussing options that did not appeal to us.

"Chemo and radiation will only weaken him further," Rick argued.

"There is something else we could try," Dr. Grana smiled.

Our posture straightened. The fact that there was anything else energized us.

"What is it?" I asked.

"It's a fairly new procedure called autologous stem cell rescue."

I didn't know what it was, but anything that ended with the word *rescue* didn't sound good.

"What is that?" Rick asked.

She explained, "It involves removing some of Robby's bone marrow, harvesting the cells, and then transplanting them back into him at a later date."

That "later date" would follow seven days of lethal doses of chemotherapy, virtually destroying all of his bone marrow and blood. Basically the doctors would bring Robby as close to death as possible, transplant his cells back into him, and then hope like heck that it would take.

"Do you have any experience with this?" I asked her.

"We have done it many times with leukemia patients, but not with brain tumors. Robby would be the first," she stated proudly, as though we should be honored.

"Will our insurance cover any of it?" Rick asked.

"Don't worry. It will all be paid for. We have ways to pay for treatments like this," she assured.

The room remained quiet while Rick and I absorbed what we'd heard. The risk? The procedure could kill Robby way before the cancer would get a chance to, and there would be a multitude of side effects. The possible benefits? Hopefully the cancer would not survive this kind of chemical bombardment, but there were no guarantees. The procedure was too new to have reliable results.

Realizing the experimental nature of what she was offering, my mind tried manipulating this option into a way out. "Dr. Grana, seriously, what are his chances of surviving?"

"Right now, he is not doing well. We estimate that he has maybe 10 percent chance of living five more years without this treatment."

The odds for Robby's survival had dropped significantly.

"I don't know," I said, shaking my head. "I don't think it's the right thing to do."

"Mr. and Mrs. Graham, your son is very ill. He does not have many options. We may not be able to help your son, but you can take comfort in knowing that we will learn a great deal from him to help another child someday."

I couldn't believe my ears. The doctors were writing him off and expected us to follow suit. Did they really expect me to hand my baby over to be their guinea pig? "Someday" was too far away, and I wasn't interested in saving another child right now. I needed to save my own.

We were being pressured into a decision that we weren't prepared to make. After all of the mishaps during our first week, I questioned their ability to do anything for him. I knew the torment he would have to endure if he received this treatment and could only imagine what Robby would look like after that kind of physical abuse. I couldn't do that to him, especially if they weren't convinced that it had any chance to cure him.

"We need a second opinion before we make a decision," I finally responded, hoping to buy us more time.

"There is a group of doctors in North Carolina," she said, "who specialize in these kinds of cases. I will make a few calls and see if we can arrange for you to meet with them."

I was suspicious of anyone she would refer us to, but agreed to it, hoping these other doctors would be different. It wouldn't hurt to talk to them.

A few hours later, my mother came to visit. I told her about our meeting and that the doctors didn't have any hope for Robby.

"Let's go down to St. Mary's. We can light a candle and pray," Mom suggested.

I didn't want to go. The meeting with Dr. Grana had destroyed all my energy. "I'm tired, Mom."

"Come on, it'll make you feel better."

"Maybe later."

"I've been going down there almost every day. You need to go. Come on."

I knew she wasn't going to give up. "All right, let's get this over with," I said, rolling my eyes as we left.

It was extremely hot outside, with humidity at a high. The sun shone down brightly on us. To many, I'm sure it was a beautiful day, but I would've preferred a dark, gloomy day to match the way I felt inside. On our way to the cathedral a few blocks away, Mom decided to give me a pep talk.

I faded in and out of her lecture, absorbed in my own thoughts. I was stuck in a nightmare and wanted desperately to wake from it. *Why did this have to happen? Why don't the doctors have answers?* I wanted Robby to take a magic pill and be cured, but the medicine they were offering wasn't magical, and it wouldn't necessarily make him well. There had to be a better way. Somewhere there had to be an answer.

How will our family ever recover from this? Where is God in this? I'm a good person. Robby is certainly good. He's just a little boy. What has he ever done to deserve this? My thoughts continued blocking out my mother's words.

The short walk seemed to take forever. My eyes wanted to sleep and my heart was heavy. It was a challenge simply to lift my legs. I wanted to go home, but something inside prompted me to continue on.

"You merely have to keep thinking positive," Mom's voice interrupted my thoughts. "You know I was reading this book the other day . . ." she continued as my thoughts took over again.

Life was different now, all of my hopes and dreams gone. Yet I couldn't shake the feeling that somehow things were going to improve. It didn't make sense. Robby's condition was deteriorating and the doctors didn't have much hope. My husband was camped out at Robby's bedside, insistent on being prepared for the worst, while family and friends tried to prepare me for the inevitable.

We arrived at the church in time to save me from Mom's continued barrage of pep, which was becoming difficult to endure. I squinted, the bright sun glaring in my eyes, as I reached to open the heavy wooden door to the church. Inside, we stood in the foyer for a moment while our eyes adjusted to the dim lighting. I noticed a tall statue of Jesus to my left, with several candles lit at His feet. Directly ahead, my eyes scanned the pew-covered sanctuary. The walls were adorned with stained-glass windows; the sweet smell of incense hung heavy in the air.

Awkwardly, I followed Mom through an archway leading to the back of the church, not knowing what to do. I went to church on Sundays and holidays only. I'd never come just to pray.

As we walked further inside, statues of various saints lined against the back wall came into view. Mom named each one, reciting what they were patron saint of. I recognized some from past teachings, but most were foreign to me. Mom dropped her candle into the glass holder in front of one and began to pray.

Unsatisfied with the options before me, my eyes swept the church, surveying all of the potential places to light my candle and pray. I shook my head no as each prospect crossed my view. *I don't have time for this*, I thought to myself. *I need help . . . big help.*

Then I remembered the statue of Jesus near the door. *I'm going straight to the top,* I thought as I made my way to Jesus.

The statue towered over me. I stood gazing up into His eyes. I knew it was a statue, but there was something so real about little me looking up to Him. His large painted eyes looked lovingly down upon me, making it easy for me to picture Him feeling my pain.

The glass holder clanked loudly as I dropped the candle in. Once it was lit, I again gazed up into His eyes and silently prayed. *"Dear Lord . . . I need you. Robby needs you. You're the only one who could possibly have any answers. No one else does. How are we going to get through this? Why do I feel like everything is going to be all right? Am I crazy? Is it really possible or just fantasy?"*

Tears began to stream down my face. *"Oh Lord, Robby's not doing very well. He can't move. He can't talk. His days are filled with pain,"* I began to cry harder as I listed all of Robby's challenges. *"God, it hurts me so much to see him this way. What am I going to do?"* I sobbed, crying uncontrollably, my face in my hands.

Suddenly, from behind, a comforting grasp came upon my right shoulder. The unseen person leaned in, as a calming voice whispered in my right ear, "Shhhh."

The flow of tears ceased. My head lifted from my hands as my eyes locked onto His. Pleasurable warmth poured over the top of my head. Difficult to describe, the feeling was tender and loving, while also strong and powerful. Calming peace accompanied its movement through my body and spirit. Slowly it flowed as honey, covering me like a cozy blanket.

"Lord . . . is that you?" I asked. My heart was racing. Was Jesus standing behind me? I was afraid to look. The hand remained firmly on my shoulder.

"Everything will be all right," the powerful whisper confirmed. "Your son will be fine. Just do what I tell you to do."

"Do? What do I need to do? I responded.

I could no longer feel the presence around me. As quickly as the encounter began, it was over. Courageously I looked over my right shoulder. There was no one there. My head jolted to the left. Nothing but the exit.

Was someone playing a trick on me? If so, they couldn't have left out that door. The foyer was dimly lit and the sun would have beamed in noticeably, I rationalized. I quickly turned again to the right, looking around the sanctuary. An elderly woman sat in one of the pews praying. Mom was still praying in the back of the church.

I saw no light beaming from the heavens. No choir of angels singing, but I absolutely knew what I heard and what I felt. Yet apparently no one else had seen or heard anything.

I looked back up at Jesus. "Lord, tell me what to do." I whispered.

No reply.

"Just tell me and I'll do it!" I prayerfully demanded.

I didn't know when or how, but a knowing in my heart confirmed He would show me what to do when it was time. Everything *was* going to be okay.

Suddenly Mom was standing behind me. "Are you ready?" she asked.

I turned to her and smiled, "Yes, I'm ready."

As we exited, my eyes burned from the brightness of the sun. The pep talk resumed.

Oh brother, I don't need to hear this, I thought. Then it became clear. *She doesn't realize what happened.* How could I tell her? I couldn't, not now. Nor could I tell anyone, for that matter. Who would ever believe me? People were already saying I was in denial. If I shared this, they would certainly think I was out of touch with reality. *For now, I'll keep this to myself.*

"Mom, everything is going to be alright," I said aloud. "I can't explain it to you, but I know that everything is going to work out. Robby is going to be fine," I oozed enthusiastically.

"I know he is. That's what I keep trying to tell you. You've got to keep thinking positive and tell him to look forward to things when he goes home. That's what I've been doing . . ."

On and on she went. I continued in my thoughts as Mom persisted. I had so much energy, I felt like I would explode. My pace increased, even skipping at times, down the sidewalk.

Mom smiled. "Slow down," she chided, her look indicating my behavior was strange.

Peace that passes all understanding, joy unspeakable, I had heard of these things, but now I knew what it meant. I felt fantastic as I nearly flew back toward the hospital.

"Come on, Mom, hurry up. I have to get back to the hospital and tell Robby that he's going to be alright!"

At the hospital entrance, Mom said good-bye, and then I continued inside. With great purpose, I walked swiftly toward the elevators. Suddenly I came to an immediate stop as the voice began to speak again. It wasn't audible this time—more like a whisper in my heart. Staff and visitors walked by with questioning looks as I stood motionless in the middle of the hall, listening intently.

"The work is done here. There's something else."

"What? What else is there? I know of nothing else, but if there is something I'll gladly go; just tell me where," I prayed silently.

Again . . . no answer, why couldn't He just tell me everything?

Riding the elevator up to Robby's room, I thought to myself. *Great! How on earth am I going to explain this? How do I tell Rick that we're supposed to go somewhere else?* I imagined the ridiculous conversation. It scared me. Now *I* was starting to think I was crazy.

Then His words rang again in my ears, *"Do what I tell you to do."*

"There has to be a way to do this without people getting in my way. Lord, please show me how to get Robby out of here, what to say, and who to say it to." I prayed. Exiting the elevator on the second floor, I focused on telling Robby that he was going to get better.

Robby was lying in bed watching television. He didn't move much anymore except when he cried. My once energetic, full-of-life child was now a depressed, almost lifeless, shell of a human being.

Rick was sitting next to him, leaning over the side rail. I hurt for my husband and longed to make him feel better too. Here was a man, normally clean and neat, who was no longer concerned about himself. His hair was disheveled, his face covered with bristles, approaching his first beard. Darkness circled beneath his bloodshot eyes. His clothes were all wrinkled and he looked as exhausted as he probably felt. He hadn't been sleeping or eating any more than I—probably less. It was a pathetic sight. This man who dedicated his life to rescuing people from dark places was now in need of rescue himself.

"Hello!" I chimed as I walked in the door, grinning uncontrollably from ear to ear.

Robby didn't move. Rick glanced up at me. I could see he was angry. (I later found out another doctor had been in while I was gone and told him more things that he didn't want to hear.)

I bent over to kiss Robby on the cheek. Rick sat up a little more now, looking at me rather puzzled. From the opposite side of the bed, I leaned over.

"Everything's going to be alright," I whispered, still grinning uncontrollably.

Now he looked at me like I was crazy.

"What?" he asked.

"Everything is going to be alright," I repeated.

He stared at me a moment, beginning to look intrigued. "How do you know?" he asked sarcastically.

I hesitated for a moment, deciding whether or not to tell him.

I continued to smile. "God told me," I whispered back.

He looked at me as if part of him thought I had lost my mind, but another part wanted it to be true.

"God told you?" he asked, sarcasm still filling his voice.

"Yep," I answered, smiling.

He continued to press on with more questions.

"Something amazing happened to me at the church . . . but I don't know if I should tell you now. You'll have to trust me."

Curiosity had the best of him. "Tell me!" he demanded.

I proceeded to give him testimony of what had happened.

"So, what are we supposed to do?" he asked.

"Well . . . there's something else."

"What do you mean 'something else'?"

I shrugged my shoulders. "We're supposed to take him somewhere else."

"Where?"

I paused for a moment trying to decide how best to tell him. "I don't know."

"What do you mean you don't know?" His voice rose.

"Shhhh."

"You mean to tell me that God talked to you, told you to take Robby somewhere else, but He didn't say where?" He asked, beginning to get overwrought.

"Yep."

"What kind of crap is that?" he asked.

"I don't know where, but He said, *'Do what I tell you to,'* so I guess He'll tell us where to go when He's ready."

Rick shrugged his shoulders, sinking into his chair, clearly annoyed. He was definitely not as excited as I. How could I expect him to be? After all, I was the one who was given a glimpse of light in the middle of darkness. At the depth of my being, I could feel God's refuge as He held us in the palm of His hand. I'd been blessed by an encounter with the Great Physician, and I would never be the same.

6
NAVIGATION

In the late fifteenth century, a man dared to believe the vision on his heart, determined to follow destiny. In a time when human beings were tied to stakes and set ablaze, independent minds were considered dangerous. The smell of burning flesh filled the air, a reminder of the penalty for thinking differently from those in authority. Dreamers were discouraged, but this navigator was compelled to prove that the Earth indeed was round and the ocean small enough to cross. When the world looked onto the ocean, they saw the impossible. When Christopher Columbus looked upon the vast seas, he saw a route to the Indies.

Armed with a strong faith, he set sail, leaving the known world behind. Many obstacles lay ahead, but he knew exactly where he was going and believed he would get there . . .

So did I.

Radio waves filled the car with sad songs while the lonely ride home toyed with my emotions. Only the passing flash of street lights penetrated the darkness as I drove. Staring into the distance, barely attentive to the trail of red lights in front of me, my eyes watered as Mariah Carey sweetly sang, "Never had I imagined, living without your smile . . . "[1] I poked the buttons on the radio. My effort to find a better song betrayed as Sarah McLachlan crooned, "I will remember you. Will you remember me?"[2]

I suppressed the melancholy feelings that tried to arise, determined that this night would be different. I pulled into my mother-in-law's driveway, not surprised that the lights were out. *Good, the kids are asleep,* I thought to myself.

Sharron, Rick's mom, greeted me at the door. "Another late night, huh?" she whispered.

"Yes. I'm sorry, but we had an eventful day." I exploded with enthusiasm. "This doctor from North Carolina called Rick." I was psyched. This had to be God's "somewhere else." "He's the chief of pediatric neuro-oncology at Duke University. Rick was really impressed with him. As soon as Robby is strong enough, we're going to take him there for a second opinion."

Reluctant to participate in my optimism, she was eager to share something of her own. "Here," she said, handing me a stack of folded papers.

"What's this?"

"One of my customers gave it to me. Read it. I think it can help Robby."

I loved my mother-in-law dearly and I knew her heart was in the right place, but she was a waitress in a mom-and-pop restaurant. What could her customer come up with that some of the world's best doctors couldn't? We already had our answer—in North Carolina. The solution was obvious. God was sending us to the right place. I wasn't interested in reading whatever she was handing me. But I knew she would pressure me until I agreed, and I was too tired to argue.

Though cynical of any usefulness, I halfheartedly accepted. "Okay, I'll read it later."

I carried Ricky and Amanda into the van and headed home. Once there, after tucking the kids in bed, I considered repeating my latest nightly ritual. I usually called my sister-in-law Christine to give her an update on Robby and talk for a couple of hours. Then, most nights, I would spend another hour or two reading about medulloblastoma, searching for answers in my Bible, or watching inspirational programs. I'd go until I passed out, and when the alarm went off in the morning, I'd start again.

But tonight, I needed to write down the numerous questions I had for Dr. Friedman at Duke. It was difficult keeping track of all the advice we were getting, so we'd begun recording our questions in a spiral notebook, adding their answers as acquired.

Attempting to relax, I laid down to watch TV, but the paper Sharron had given me kept calling me. I tried ignoring it. I was tired and needed to sleep, but I couldn't stop glancing down to the floor where I'd tossed the newsletter on my way in.

"I'll read it tomorrow," I told myself, rolling over in time to watch Steve Irwin jump bravely onto another croc. I was in awe of him, but he was competing with a stronger force. My attention was distracted yet again, drawn to the short stack of paper on the floor. Something kept prompting me to read it. Unable to withstand it any longer, I snatched up the newsletter and began reading.

"Everyone's Health Is at Stake If We Lose This Therapy," the headline read.[3]

My eyes scanned the eight-page newsletter, searching for something that pertained to me.

"In February 1994, two-and-a-half-year-old Dustin Kunnari was diagnosed with medulloblastoma . . . "[4] Aha. "They refused chemotherapy and radiation." *Hmmm, how did they do that?* I wondered.

The article went on to say that their doctor advised them to do the same things our doctors were advising us, citing a success rate of 20–40 percent. "Yet they could not name a single patient on whom the program had been successful." The doctor told them ". . . she hoped Dustin would be alive in five years, but he could be in a wheelchair, and would have stunted growth and learning disabilities."[5]

Oh God, these are the things I fear. I knew that the side effects of chemo and radiation were significant, especially at the high doses necessary for treating the brain.

"Doctors Threatened to Take Them to Court."[6]

"That's not fair!" I argued aloud with the newsletter.

"The Kunnaris quickly researched alternatives and decided to give Burzynski's treatment a try. . . . They began Antineoplaston therapy in April 1994, and in six weeks the MRI showed complete remission."[7]

Awesome! But what is this Antineoplaston therapy? I wondered as I continued reading.

The article was compelling. Just like me, these people didn't want themselves or their loved ones to be incapacitated by the very treatment meant to save their lives. There was also a story about a four-year-old girl, the same age as Robby, who lost her battle—not because of the cancer but as a result of the conventional therapy she had received.

Her father wrote, "I will never be able to communicate what we put Cryssie through. The horrible sickness from her chemotherapy and radiation made her so ill, most of us would have given up our lives just from the pain. We stole her hair, her sight, and in the end her ability to walk and talk."[8] Her parents wanted people to know that there was something available other than what conventional medicine had to offer.

The Antineoplaston treatment, discovered and developed by Dr. Burzynski, was a synthetic version of a set of amino acids found in the human body. It could be administered orally or by IV and was considered to be nontoxic and relatively side-effect free.

Could this be true? Was there really a nontoxic chemotherapy treatment available in the United States? Could it work for Robby? How would we pay for it? I wanted this. Now I was torn, my excitement about North Carolina short-lived. Was Houston the place God wanted us to go?

Inspired by the film *Lorenzo's Oil,* a movie about parents who found a cure for the incurable illness that plagued their son,[9] I decided to learn all I could about my son's disease and anything that might cure it. My passion ignited, I spent several nights on friends' computers doing my own research. The Internet was still fairly new, making it difficult to learn anything substantive about the disease, even more difficult to discover treatment options.

At one site, a well-known medical library provided excerpts of research publications. The information therein was not appealing, however. These reports, filed by some of the same experts who wanted to treat my son, lacked anything positive to say. The results they reported, achieved with the same modalities of treatment our doctors were trying hard to sell us on, were minimal at best.

A study from Cambridge Hospital, dated March 1997, read: "Recurrent medulloblastoma has long been considered universally fatal. In spite of attempts to improve its treatment, only rarely have long-term survivors been documented in the world's medical literature. Although the treatment of primary medulloblastoma is well established and includes surgical excision, postsurgical irradiation, and, more recently, chemotherapy, there is no established treatment for its recurrence."[10] Hopefully we wouldn't ever have to deal with recurrence. What about treatment for the initial diagnosis?

There were plenty of medications being investigated with adults, but none for children. The disease my son was fighting primarily affected children, but most of the drugs and treatments offered were tested only on adults with totally different cancers. Still, the link to Dr. Burzynski appeared in every search I tried, and it seemed to be the only possibility for a child. The more I learned, the less I knew what to do. I teetered back and forth between the course offered by the conventional specialists at Duke, and Dr. Burzynski's therapy.

"Lord, I want to try this treatment in Houston," I prayed, *"but we need to go where You want. Please, show us which way to go. We can't afford to pay for this treatment, and our insurance won't pay either. If this is the place . . . then please, please send the money . . . quickly,"* I pleaded. *"If the money comes, we'll know this is the way to go. If not, then we'll keep moving forward until You reveal the next step."*

Two long weeks passed. I thought by now things would've improved. Yet Robby hadn't eaten since surgery, his tiny body dwindling away. Finally the medical staff decided they should do something about it, wanting to insert a feeding tube.

I refused. They were convinced it was the right thing to do. I, on the other hand, was not. The vivid memory of a tube pushed down my nose and throat six months earlier reminded me of the pain of my own deadly illness. Images flashed in my mind: the feel of the cold steel as the doctor pierced my back to sample the unknown mass inside . . . the taste of barium after all ten CT scans . . . troubled looks on the faces of family and friends.

Disturbing memories came flooding back. The untold hours spent alone, lying in the hospital bed, crying. My body convulsed with constant vomiting and diarrhea, the stabbing pain from my gut was unbearable. I felt hopeless as my body swelled up with fluid, my organs shutting down. My soul was clinging to life, while my body was letting it slip away.

Now it was my little boy who was suffering. I couldn't bear the thought of putting him through more torture. I also knew that once a tube was inserted, it could be very difficult to get it removed. Robby already had a Mediport. Why couldn't they use that?

Most of the day was spent trying to convince the dietician to see things my way. Exhausted with the debate, she finally asked Robby's intensive care doctor to speak with me. Though Robby was no longer in ICU, the doctor continued to follow his case.

Subsequently, the doctor and I argued the pros and cons of a feeding tube. I told him of my experience, and he assured me that children were different. I expressed every fear, but he had an answer for each one.

"We're certain that if we get something into his stomach, he'll automatically begin to want food," the doctor explained.

Again I countered. "I'm certain that he's simply weak, and if you'll give him the IV nutrition, he'll get strong enough to eat."

They had given Robby a chart to communicate with. On it were pictures of Mom and Dad, food and drink, pain, and the potty. He had already been pointing to the picture of food for days, but they wouldn't let him eat because of his swallowing difficulty.

The doctor continued, "If we put the nutrition through the Mediport it could get clogged, and then he'll have to have surgery to replace it. Do you want to put him through another operation?"

No, I didn't want to take that chance either. Reluctantly, I agreed.

"I promise I'll put it in myself," he assured me.

Robby cried and swung at them with his one little moving arm. His two right limbs flailed in an attempt to get away. A few moments later the tube was in. As the doctor left the room, he stopped near me and said, "You did the right thing." He smiled and walked out.

At Robby's side, the nurse was finishing what the doctor started. The feeding tube needed to be anchored with tape, but before she could get it on, the tube had all but fallen out. As she tried to push it back down, Robby gagged and cried. Now it was stuck in the back of his throat. She tried to pull it out. Robby screamed with pain. Now the tip was stuck in his nose.

I stood there watching, my arms crossed, daggers flying out of my eyes. Another nurse came in to help, but it was stuck. Robby wailed in agony. The doctor was called to return. Surely he knew I was furious. I stood posed in the same stance—my arms crossed, my foot now tapping on the floor. One of the nurses put her arm around me as the doctor pulled and twisted, and my son cried even more.

"I know this isn't easy for you," she said.

"I didn't want this anyway!" I snapped through clenched teeth.

Her arm quickly dropped from my shoulders. Finally the tube was out.

The doctor glanced toward me. Then, looking to the ground, he solemnly agreed. "I'll order the IV nutrition."

I was pleased, until several hours later when we were told that the solution had to be mixed by the pharmacist, who had gone home. My little pumpkin would have to stay hungry another day.

Twenty-four hours later, the IV nutrition began. A day after that, Robby was eating.

"I've never seen anything like it!" the dietician exclaimed.

Normally it takes several days for a patient to begin eating full meals after the stomach has been empty for nearly two weeks, but he was eating entire meals and then some.

Robby's energy level began to increase and his disposition improved. Of course, he still played possum whenever the nurses and doctors came in to check him. He didn't like that. But when alone, we were beginning to see some of the real Robby coming back. His big brother, Ricky, began to visit more and Robby loved it. His mood was significantly elevated when Ricky visited. Something special about his big brother inspired him.

During one of Ricky's visits, Robby slowly exclaimed, "Rrrr-iiiiiii-cky!" We were thrilled, thinking he had finally begun to talk again, but it was the only word he said. After that, his silence continued.

"Knock, knock." Mike's smiling face peeked through the doorway.

Rick and Robby lay on the hospital bed, while I leaned back in a nearby chair, all of us lethargic from staring at endless hours of cartoons.

"Come on in," Rick said.

Mike was a district chief at Rick's fire department. He was a soft-spoken man, a committed husband and father, and a regular giver in the community. He was also a hard worker with a lot on his plate.

It was nice to have a visitor. The atmosphere in the room needed brightening—even a brief touch of outside light helped. He asked how we were doing, and we filled him in on our two prospects for treatment.

"Listen . . . uh . . . we've been talking, at the department, about what we can do to help you guys out."

"You don't have to do that, Mike," Rick replied.

Sensitive to Rick's ego, not wanting to embarrass or insult him, Mike encouraged Rick to receive their gift. "Even with two insurance plans you're bound to have expenses that aren't covered. Please, let us do this. It's not much, but it'll help."

"What did you have in mind?" I asked.

"Well, the guys were talking about having a car wash, and we've got a couple other ideas. Several people have stepped up and said they're prepared to make donations, and it looks like a few businesses might help too."

"What do you need us to do?" Rick asked.

"Don't worry. Let me take care of everything. You guys have enough to do already. You just concentrate on helping Robby get better and take care of yourselves."

I was in a much better mood after Mike's visit. "Honey, I think we're going to Houston."

"Just because they're opening an account doesn't mean there will be money in it. We need an awful lot of money to go there," he stated. Even though his response was cynical, a ray of hope began to shine in Rick's eyes.

I answered back, "Well, we'll see. All I know is that we've got to get him out of here. We're going to North Carolina. Maybe we can take him to Houston for a consult before making our decision. If the money comes by then, we'll know what we're supposed to do."

The next day I called the clinic in Houston and requested an information packet and application. Another disappointment—all patients had to be accepted into the program by meeting the protocol, and then their participation had to be approved by the FDA. I thought from what I'd read that Robby would qualify, but the waiting period was two to four weeks. There was no way the doctors would leave us alone that long to make a decision. They were already pressuring us to begin treatment. The nature of the disease was aggressive; in a month's time, we might be right back where we started. Neither of us wanted to put him through another brain surgery.

We asked the oncologists what they knew about Dr. Burzynski's treatment. They didn't know much, but were adamant that it was not the route to take. It didn't take long for us to decide to stop discussing it with them. Having your children taken away for not following medical advice was not uncommon in our town. We couldn't let that happen.

We were going for a second opinion at one of the leading medical centers in the world for treatment of pediatric brain tumors. That was one thing the local doctors couldn't argue against, although they did tell us they could do the exact same protocol here. Somehow that didn't impress us—especially after they performed the spinal tap that Dr. Friedman explicitly said was contraindicated.

Did they really write his instructions on a yellow sticky note? No wonder it was ignored. How many of their mistakes could we survive?

Moreover, I was trying to build an army. Not just any army, but one that could win. My son needed to have the best, and from what I understood, the doctors at Duke fit that requirement. They were the most experienced and, logically, the ones to trust. I didn't know how this was all going to come together, but it would.

After twenty days in the hospital, Robby was finally going home. During his hospital stay, he'd consistently refused the wheelchair, riding only in a wagon or Daddy's arms. He hated wheelchairs, but now he was going home with one. It was specially ordered for his miniature body. The tiny chair was brand-new, equipped with a reclining back since he couldn't sit up on his own. His left eye remained severely crossed, his ability to talk hadn't yet returned.

I thought he would be eager to go home, but there was no evidence of that. Upon our arrival, we eagerly showed Robby his new bed. I had purchased two juvenile-sized air mattresses for the boys to camp out in the living room. I thought it would be fun for them, and I didn't want him sleeping in his own bed. He might fall out and hurt himself.

Yet being home did not ignite the magic for Robby that I thought it would. He would lie on his mattress all day watching Ricky, uninterested in playing along. Waves of doubt crashed upon me. But we had already navigated many obstacles, and I had a certainty in my heart that we were on the right path. God was still opening doors to possibilities I had yet to discover. Despite the depth of the unknown, I held tightly to my vision for Robby's healing. After all, I was compelled to follow destiny.

7
PRECISION

She was the greatest ship ever to have been built. Thousands of carpenters, engineers, master mechanics, electricians, painters, decorators, and the like fitted this vessel with the latest in marine technology and the finest decor. This mechanical marvel was assembled with precision and fine craftsmanship, crewed by highly trained men and women prepared to serve the elite. Loaded with both reciprocating steam engines and a turbine engine to power three gigantic propellers, no other could compete. The double-plated hull housed a sophisticated system of sixteen watertight compartments, providing the utmost security to both passengers and crew. She was unsinkable.[1]

With the past three weeks' experience behind us, I had a renewed appreciation for skill and accuracy. Looking forward to meeting Dr. Friedman at Duke, I hoped his knowledge and expertise would surpass all we'd recently encountered.

As the plane took off, we tried to coax Robby to look out the window. He wasn't interested, unhappy that he couldn't eat what he wanted. He leaned onto his father's arm, unable to sit up on his own. I could tell he was uncomfortable and not feeling well. Tears began to swell in my eyes. This was his first time flying. It wasn't supposed to be this way.

He should be excited and going someplace fun, I thought.

We were on our way to North Carolina, blessed to have our entire trip covered by generous donors. Our friend Guy chauffeured us to the airport in one of his stretch limos. The limousine ride was also a first for Robby, but it didn't thrill him either.

We arrived at the hotel in late afternoon. The homey, Southern-styled building was nestled cozily in a deeply wooded area off the highway. We had never stayed any place so nice. The kind stranger who provided these exquisite accommodations was greatly appreciated.

Once settled into our room, we decided to go for a drive. It felt good to be outside for a change, and the scenery was the right prescription for us. We thought getting out would lift Robby's spirits, but he didn't appreciate the big deal we made out of everything. Using a cellular phone, also donated, was a new privilege. The "brick," as it was called, was bulky and awkward, but it was a lot of fun to call Ricky from the car as we traveled the tree-lined highways of North Carolina.

Beep—beep—beep—beep. The alarm blared. I hated getting up early. Rick was an early bird. I was the night owl.

"Is it six o'clock already?" I asked, my eyes still closed.

"Yes, time to get up. I want to leave extra early so we get to the hospital on time."

While he showered, I called home to check our voice mail. It too was something new for us, forced by our present circumstance.

I had never retrieved messages over the phone before. *I hope this works*, I thought to myself.

"You have one new message," the mechanized voice reported.

"Hello, this is Kathy calling from the Burzynski Clinic. We've received your application and want to set up an appointment for Robert to come for consultation. Please give us a call back to schedule. Thank you."

Yes! I wanted to call her right back, but it was only five a.m. in Houston. As soon as I heard the shower stop, I hollered to Rick about the message, but he seemed less than enthused.

While waiting for Rick to finish getting ready, Robby and I waited patiently.

"Robby, would you like to try and stand up?" I asked.

His half-crooked smile and outstretched arms indicated a yes. I sat him on the edge of the bed, grasping both of his hands. He pushed with one leg while I pulled on both arms, holding him in a standing position, like an infant learning to walk.

Maybe I shouldn't have pushed him so hard, but I wanted to help him get better as fast as possible. At home, he had begun to crawl. He looked like a little wounded soldier shimmying across the floor on both elbows, pushing with one leg. He tried and tried, wanting so desperately to walk again. I just had to help free him from that wheelchair.

"Robby," I smiled, "get ready to stand."

Oh God, please don't let him fall and get hurt, I thought to myself, hoping I wasn't going to cause more harm than good. Nervous, I slowly released my hands from his.

"Robby, you did it! You're standing! Rick, get the camera!"

This was the first time in over a month that Robby was standing. He had the biggest smile, the only one I had seen since before his surgery. While I was ecstatic for him, at the same time my heart ached on his behalf. His little body was hunched over to one side. He grinned a big half-faced grin. The distortion of his cute little face, with one side paralyzed, was a reminder of the distance he still had to travel.

Rick quickly grabbed the camera and snapped our picture before Robby began to fall against the bed. I was standing near enough to catch him. He couldn't stand on his own yet, but this was a good sign. It was going to be a great day.

The enormity of the Duke medical complex astonished me. The corridors of this grand campus were vast and intimidating. It was so large that we had to take a tram from the main hospital building to the outpatient building, where we were scheduled. From there, a member of the team escorted us to the Clinic—a misleading title representative only of its function. This was no regular clinic; it was larger than the average hospital. I don't think we could've found our way without our guide.

The building was a mix of contemporary architecture and old-world passageways, which Robby's wheelchair, though small, made difficult to navigate. We followed through winding hallways, up the stairs and down the elevator, around too many corners to count. Would we be able to find our way out of this labyrinth?

The waiting room wasn't much to look at. Simple brown chairs lined the four drab-colored walls, accommodating people of all colors and sizes. More chairs formed rows in the middle of the room. There was a small play area with a few ragged toys tossed in the corner. By the sounds of various dialects, many had traveled great distances to come to this center of healing, just as we had. Some appeared to be doing better than us; others were worse.

"Mr. and Mrs. Graham?" asked a kind, bearded gentleman.

Rick and I nodded in unison.

"I'm John Legge," he said, reaching out his right hand. "Welcome to Duke. I'm the social worker and I'll be traveling with you today." The ceiling lights glimmered off his wire-rimmed glasses. His facial hair didn't do much to hide his youthful appearance.

"I'd like to say, 'Nice to meet you,' but I'd rather not be here," Rick responded.

The three of us laughed briefly.

"I certainly understand," John replied. "This must be Robby," he smiled, reaching out to shake Robby's hand. Robby looked at him quizzically, hesitant to trust this friendly stranger. "Follow me, I'll show you around a little and then introduce you to members of the team."

We followed John to an examination room. While waiting for "the team," we talked. He was kind and assuring, a wealth of information. Eventually another man came into the room.

John introduced us. "This is Dr. Halperin, the radiation oncologist."

He was a well-dressed man in a suit and tie, no lab coat. He too had a beard, yet his thinning brown hair and receding hairline gave witness to his age. Why were the radiation docs always the first ones we met? The thought of radiating my baby boy's brain, like a roast in a microwave, made me nauseous.

He discussed Robby's condition and possible ways to treat it, teaching us the meaning of his lingo in the process. This crew obviously functioned with great precision. They were at the forefront medically and technologically. Communication between them was thorough and exact. They had done their homework and knew everything about us. We felt as though we were finally headed in the right direction. Dr. Halperin excused himself, promising to return momentarily.

We then bounced from room to room through various stations and checkpoints. It seemed like forever, but eventually Dr. Halperin returned. We visited with him more while waiting to be introduced to the rest of the team. John came in and out occasionally, assuring us that everyone would be there soon.

"Dr. Friedman is a great doctor and an exceptional human being," Dr. Halperin assured us. "Medulloblastoma is his specialty, did you know that?" he asked.

"No, I had no idea." I answered.

"Really?" Rick asked.

"Yes. It's his passion to find a cure for medulloblastoma. He has been studying it for over a decade." Dr. Halperin oozed enthusiasm for the mystical man we had yet to meet. He continued, "He's a renowned researcher, very intelligent, yet down to earth. He's just a regular guy. If you see someone walking around here in jeans and sneakers, it's probably Henry."

John returned with a camera. "We'd like to get a picture of Robby, if that's alright."

"Sure," Rick replied.

John took Robby's picture, one for them and an extra for us. Then, finally, the entourage began. A dozen or so people came in and lined up for our viewing.

"Mr. and Mrs. Graham, this is the team," Dr. Halperin announced. "These, and a few others, are the people who are

61

working on Robby's case. We're all here to assist you in finding a cure for your son."

If parading the entire team into the room was meant to impress us, it worked! A small army of people working to help Robby was just what I was after. As I looked over each person, I recognized some of their positions, based upon their uniforms or formal dress. But one man stood out among the dresses, suits, and uniforms. In a sport shirt, faded tattered jeans, and old tennis shoes, he was difficult to place and didn't seem to belong.

Who's that clown? I thought to myself as he walked past, exiting in line with the team.

Next John took us to another floor to meet Dr. Friedman. This was the pinnacle of our trip, the reason we came. He was the man with all the answers.

Ushered into a tiny room filled with file cabinets, we sat at the small table for four in the corner by the window. John sat next to an empty chair on one side. Rick and I sat together on the other, anxiously awaiting the arrival of Dr. Friedman. Robby was next door with someone on "the team."

Moments later, that weird guy, the one wearing tattered jeans and sneakers, came in and sat next to John.

"Mr. and Mrs. Graham, this is Dr. Friedman," John introduced.

Dr. Friedman reached out to shake my hand. "Call me Henry."

My jaw dropped. I thought I was going to fall out of my chair. Rick and I glanced at each other questioningly; our eyes widened and our lips twisted.

Unsure of what to think, I was quite surprised that *this* was the doctor we had waited so impatiently to see. Why hadn't he been introduced to us downstairs? I was not impressed.

However, all of my concerns quickly dissipated as Dr. Friedman began to talk. He thoroughly educated us on the disease, all of the potential treatment modalities, and his plan for Robby's treatment. He was phenomenal. His recommendation was for radiation followed by autologous bone marrow rescue, basically the same treatment offered at home, with one huge difference—at Duke they had actually carried it off successfully more than seventy-five times.

Though I had a lot of concerns about the proposed treatment, at least here they had more experience and success. If we didn't want to travel back and forth, they could have Robby's doctors at home carry out Duke's protocol while Dr. Friedman monitored him from a distance.

We were intrigued by his impressive statistics and claims of highly successful results. He even had a name for why Robby wasn't able to talk. "It's called cerebellar mutism. That's not uncommon after surgery in that area. It usually goes away in time," he explained confidently

We were *very* impressed.

Dr. Friedman was extremely knowledgeable and optimistic. His confidence enhanced his persuasiveness. Thorough and convincing, I believed this man could sell ice to Eskimos. He was agreeable to us supplying nutritional support through vitamins and food. And he had more knowledge about supplements than any other doctor thus far.

But this was my baby we were talking about, and I wanted to make sure that we discussed *every* treatment option. So I decided to push the envelope. "What do you know about Antineoplastons?"

"Are you talking about Dr. Burzynski?" he asked, making a face that quickly indicated his disapproval.

Rick and I nodded our heads yes.

He proceeded to tell us what he knew, which was very little. "Well, from what we know, it can't hurt him, but it won't help him either. Let me rephrase that. It *can* hurt him in that if he doesn't get appropriate treatment, his disease will kill him," he stated definitively, his voice rising.

That wasn't good enough for me. I had done my homework. This man had access to medical literature that I didn't have, so surely he must know more. I pressed him with detailed questions.

Instead of answering me, Dr. Friedman stood up, rambling things about Dr. Burzynski and his treatment that were unfounded and don't bear repeating, his voice rising the entire time. He threw Robby's file down on the table and stormed out, slamming the door behind him.

Rick, John, and I exchanged wide-eyed looks of bewilderment. None of us knowing what to say, the room was silent for a moment while we processed what just happened.

Rick leaned over and whispered in my ear, "Maybe we shouldn't go to Texas."

Oh no. Now what was I going to do? Rick was obviously feeling like these were the people to get the job done, but something in me wasn't satisfied. I had to know more.

I looked intently at John as I responded. "No. He didn't answer my questions." I leaned forward on the table, my arms crossed. "You go out there," I said sternly, pointing at the door, "and tell him to get back in here."

John grinned, stood up, and exited the room. A few seconds later the two of them returned. Dr. Friedman was smiling as he pulled his chair up to the table. He calmly sat down and we began to discuss things further.

I was tired of being pushed around by all of these doctors. This wasn't a game to me, and I refused to be a pawn. It was my turn to be in charge.

"So, you basically don't know anything about it, do you?" I questioned.

Henry tried his best to answer me, but it didn't take long for me to figure things out. "We don't know much about it, except that it doesn't work," he conceded.

Rick and John remained quiet observers.

"Well, we need some time to think about what we want to do. Give us a few days and we'll let you know," I concluded.

"We'll probably be bringing him back here," Rick stated.

Dr. Friedman smiled and we said our good-byes.

Our drive back to the hotel was fairly quiet, both of us digesting the new information. One thing was certain—Rick was definitely impressed by "the team." Convincing him to remain open-minded was not going to be easy. Meanwhile, I had my own confusing thoughts to deal with. Clearly, if traditional medicine was the route we were to take, this was the place to be. It was the best of the best.

Even so, I had this unexplainable desire to investigate our options in Houston. It made no sense to my mind, yet my heart was insistent. I called Dr. Burzynski's office the first chance I got.

"Good afternoon. Burzynski Research Institute," a kind female voice answered.

"Hello, may I speak with Kathy?"

"I'm sorry, she's not available. Can I take a message?" her Southern drawl melodically asked.

"Well . . . my name is Leslie Graham. I am returning her call."

"I can take a message and have her call you back."

"Umm . . . I'm not home. I'm getting a second opinion out of state and was really hoping I could talk to someone."

"Hold on a minute, honey."

A minute or two later, she returned.

"I have your file. Your son's name is Robert, right?"

"Yes, that's right."

"We need to see you right away."

"As I said, we are in North Carolina right now. I would really like to get a few questions answered first."

She proceeded to give me details on the kind of financial commitment we would need to make, and some basics about the treatment. Of course she couldn't get too specific without the doctor evaluating the case first.

"We're really not sure what we want to do. We'd like to come there and find out what you have to offer," I told her. "But the doctors here are extremely knowledgeable and very convincing."

"I understand," she said. "I tell you, honey, before you do anything, I would surely give this a chance. I've seen those poor little babies come in here after that other stuff doesn't work, and it's terrible."

I was extremely confused. My heart could hear and feel what she was saying, but what if it was just a sales pitch? With the abundance of information we now had, I didn't know whom to believe. The only way to find out was to go there.

Why did the decision have to be so complicated? In the end, Duke had the skill and perfection we sought. There, dozens of skilled professionals worked together like a precision machine. But the pages of history revealed the dangers of having too much faith in men. Such misplaced trust can be deadly. In the case of the RMS *Titanic*, the unsinkable ship sank. I couldn't make the same mistake.

8
LIKE A CHILD

When viewed through the eyes of a child, the world is a place of wonder and amazement. As a young girl, I was always on a mission of discovery. Rare treasures of the utmost beauty and rarity could be found right in my own backyard. If I hunted well, I would find the most colorful snail or the prettiest feathers I'd ever seen. While dandelions were unwelcome guests to some, making wishes while blowing on them was always certain to bring me good fortune. Sometimes I would spend hours with friends, combing through patches of clover, lucky to find the one with four leaves. Sure, it took some time to find my riches, but it was always worth it. Quite often, the best things in life can be found right in front of us, but they can only be seen when we take the time to look.

Armed with a list of former Burzynski patients, I began making calls. Each had only good things to say, though their levels of success varied. Then I called Mariann. Her son had been treated for medulloblastoma—the same boy I had read about in the newsletter.

Dustin had no other treatment besides surgery and Antineoplastons. He had one recurrence, but they were able to induce remission again simply by boosting his dosage of this special medication. It had been two years and he was still cancer free. It sounded fantastic. Could it work for us too? I wanted it to, but we were still unsure. After talking to these families, and some further discussion between Rick and myself, we decided to go to Houston to meet Dr. Burzynski. We needed to see with our own eyes what this man really offered.

Before we could go, Robby would have to get another MRI. The doctors at Duke thought the MRI of Robby's spine was done too soon following surgery, indicating a possible false reading. The cancer may not have spread to his spine after all.

On our way to the MRI appointment, I laid my hands on Robby's back and prayed for God to intervene: "They don't even know if anything is really there or not," I prayed, "so please, God, if there is, just make it go away."

We received Robby's MRI results the evening before our scheduled flight to Houston. The report read, "Apparent resolution of extensive abnormal signal in the thoracolumbar thecal sac compared with previous exam. Therefore, this does not appear to represent metastatic disease given the short time interval and the lack of intervening therapy since the previous study." In short, there was no cancer in his spine. I didn't care what they thought or what was there before—I was just glad it was gone.

In Dr. Burzynski's parking lot, we sat silently, our eyes fixed on the place for which we held high expectations. This two-story office building was dwarfed by the memory of the mammoth complex we visited the week before. There was no comparison.

Rick pushed Robby's wheelchair as we ventured into the lobby. On board the elevator, loud squeaking noises screeched as we began to rise. Rick looked up toward the sound. Then he nudged Robby on the shoulder. "Hey Robby . . . sounds like they've got the squirrels working this thing."

We all chuckled.

I nodded my head and smiled. *Well, at least his sense of humor is beginning to make an appearance again,* I thought silently.

The elevator doors opened to the second floor, revealing a large sign upon the wall.

BURZYNSKI RESEARCH INSTITUTE, INC.
Administrative Offices

S.R. BURZYNSKI, MD, PhD
CLINIC

"This is it. Are you ready?" Rick asked.

I nodded my head yes and we both took a deep breath as I opened the door.

The waiting area was unlike any other we'd visited. Instead of the sterile, lifeless environment hosted by most health care providers, this one implored you to come in and take a look around. The spacious yet cozy room housed several big, cushy leather sofas. A home entertainment center on one wall housed a large television. In a nearby corner, a video game table sat surrounded by brightly colored toys. All of this, combined with the personal photographs on the walls, gave the comfortable feeling of home.

The faces of great men—Albert Einstein, Louis Pasteur, and Pope John Paul II among them—also graced the walls. I gazed around the room, and then noticed the reception window with a large cross hanging directly above it. This place was different.

We handed our records and MRI copies through the window, and in return received a clipboard with more papers to fill out. I was used to that by now.

We sat down in the cozy room as we waited for our appointment. Before long we were happily greeted.

"Hello, is this Robert?" a smiling, young lady asked. Her tan Latino skin and wavy black hair glowed in unison with her smile.

"Yes," Rick and I answered.

"Hi. I'm Gabriella. Please, come with me."

We followed her to a room close by.

"Please have a seat and be comfortable," she requested.

Rick and I sat side by side, opposite Gabriella. Robby's wheelchair fit nicely by the side of the desk.

Gabriella noticed the red yarn necklace with a large wooden cross that Robby wore. He'd made it at school and insisted on wearing it.

"Do you know Jesus?" she asked Robby.

Robby nodded his head yes.

She said emphatically, "I know Him too! I love Him very much. He's very good to us."

Rick and I smiled approvingly.

I love this place, I thought to myself.

Gabriella reviewed page upon page of government notices regarding the risks of treatment in a clinical trial, as well as their financial charges and payment policies. The initial start-up cost was $14,000. The medication alone was $5,000 a month, plus charges for supplies, labs, etc., and we would need to buy the IV pump.

Rick shook his head as we heard the numbers. "Does insurance cover any of that?"

"Some do, but most do not because it is an experimental medication," Gabriella answered. "We don't file insurance right now, so you will have to pay and then get reimbursed by your insurance."

I could tell by the glare Rick gave me that he didn't think it would ever happen. I didn't care. I wasn't going to let money get in my way. If this were the right place to be, I'd find a way to pay.

Next we met some of the nurses who took vitals, blood work, and so on. Conversations with most of the staff we met were laced with references to God. I was impressed and relieved. It was refreshing to be in a professional place where the staff felt comfortable mentioning the name of Jesus.

We expected this would be a brief appointment. After all, how long could it take to get an evaluation? Back in the waiting area again, we grew to appreciate the comfortable seating. As the day marched on, the lobby became more and more crowded. Office staff and nurses buzzed busily around.

A number of other people waited also, some sicker than others. Many appeared defeated in their attempts at conventional medicine, now giving their last hope to this treatment. There were people of all ages, but mostly adults. The majority toted backpacks or fanny packs, IV tubes flowing out from under their clothing.

Some were happy and energetic. Others . . . well, they seemed happy to just be alive.

After several hours, we were finally called into one of the patient rooms. There we waited some more.

Eventually a woman entered, wearing glasses and clothed in a white lab coat. "Hello. I'm Dr. Rita," she smiled, extending her hand, shaking ours.

She was new to the facility, and in training. She did her best to answer our questions while examining Robby. As we quizzed her, it was clear that she wanted to give us hope, but for reasons unknown, she was holding back. She finished her examination and announced that Dr. Burzynski would soon be in.

Half an hour later, the door opened again.

"Hello. I'm Dr, Burzynski," he announced with a strong Polish accent as he walked in smiling.

He examined Robby quickly, noticeably less comprehensive than Dr. Rita. I assumed he was looking at specifics, since she had already performed a thorough physical. Rick, sitting behind him, made sure I saw his facial expressions, clearly not approving.

"We can enter him in protocol," Dr. Burzynski informed us.

"Can you tell us more about the treatment?" I asked.

"Certainly."

"We've read that it is not toxic."

"This is true," he replied.

"How many children have you treated?" Rick asked.

"Oh, I have many patients who are children."

"And they all had medulloblastoma?" I asked, to clarify.

"No, no, they are all different."

"How many kids with medulloblastoma have you treated?"

"I have treated only four," he answered.

Not the best statistics to make a decision by. I questioned his numbers. "Only four? Did it work for all of them?"

"No. Two are in remission, one unchanged, and one died."

Robby was hungry and beginning to get very agitated.

"Could you give us a few minutes to discuss this alone?" I asked.

"Sure. I'll be back in a little while," the doctor answered.

Once the door was closed, Rick said, "What in the heck was he saying? Between the echo in the room and his accent, I couldn't understand a word." He was clearly agitated too. "Did he say he only treated four kids with medulloblastoma?" Rick drilled.

"Yes."

"And only two got better?" His face indicated his disgust.

"That's what he said."

"We're getting out of here. I've had enough!"

"Honey, please, I don't want to leave. Can't we at least see what else he has to say?"

My heart was breaking. Leaving meant we had to face the only other options—chemo and radiation. My eyes pleaded with him to stay.

"Alright, I'll give him one more try, but I think we should leave."

Dr. Burzynski returned a few minutes later. Rick asked a few more questions, obviously frustrated with the answers.

Finally the doctor made our options clear. "You have very difficult decision to make. The treatment might help him, or it might not. In about six weeks we will know if treatment is working. But in six weeks, if not working, you could be back where you started and he may need another surgery."

This man was a scientist. Everything he said was in a scientific, factual manner. He was not a suave salesman, like some of the other doctors we'd seen. His heavy accent didn't help either. Rick had a thing about people coming to this country and he felt that all of them should learn to speak English like any other American.

"Let me know when you make decision and we will proceed," Dr. Burzynski instructed us.

Rick was not a happy camper. He went directly to the front desk and requested all of the materials we had brought. I wanted to cry. I couldn't believe this was how things were going to end here.

"I'm out of here!" Rick emphatically declared. "I can't believe we wasted time and money to come all this way for him to tell us that it might help or it might not!"

The thought of Robby having another brain surgery was more than either of us could bear.

"I know. But I don't think we should leave yet. Can't we just think about it?" I begged, my heart winning out over my head.

"I doubt Robby can survive another brain surgery, and I don't want to play around with his life. Let's just go back to Duke."

While we were in North Carolina, I was confident of their ability to help us, but at what cost? Torturing Robby and leaving him with a life of pain and sickness wasn't an option for me. I understood where Rick was coming from, but I felt that at least treatment with Antineoplastons offered hope, and I wasn't ready to give up yet.

On our way to the exit, Dr. Rita walked by and smiled. "See you later."

"No, you won't," Rick snapped.

She looked puzzled. Clearly anyone fortunate enough to be accepted for treatment in their protocol took it. "Why are you leaving?" she asked.

I didn't say a thing, my eyes begging her to talk some sense into Rick.

"You have to understand," she said, "Dr. Burzynski is under strict observation right now and has to be careful what he says. All I can tell you is that this treatment offers the best hope."

We knew there were some issues with the government and Dr. Burzynski, but weren't clear about them. It didn't seem to matter because our use of his medicine was in an FDA-approved clinical trial.

"Well, we'll think about it," he replied.

An awkward silence accompanied us on the ride to the hotel. Back in the room, we discussed our options again. Rick would tell me why he didn't want to use this therapy, and I would beg him to pray about it before making a decision.

Lying on the bed, holding his head in his hands, Rick's fingers ran repeatedly through every hair. "I don't know what to do. I don't want to put him through chemo and radiation, but I don't want to do this either. I just want him to be well!" he shouted.

I understood what he was feeling. Our little boy's life was in our hands. What if we made the wrong choice? Why wasn't God telling us what to do?

"Honey, why don't you call Mariann?" I encouraged.

"Who's that?" he asked.

"She's the lady I talked to. You know, the mom of the boy in that newsletter."

"How am I going to do that?"

"I have her number somewhere in this stuff," I said, referring to the notebook of papers I had collected.

I couldn't believe it, but Rick called right then and there. He asked dozens of questions, for which she appeared to have the right answers.

"Feel better?" I asked.

"I feel better about the treatment. It really helped her son. But I don't know. I'm confused. I don't know what to think."

"Should I call the clinic and enroll?" I asked.

"No. Not yet."

"Ok," I conceded, disappointed.

We sat in silence, wrapped in our thoughts.

Finally I spoke again. "We have to do something. The doctors aren't going to let us go on forever without choosing something," I urged Rick.

"I know, but I don't know what to do."

"Why don't we go home and pray about it and see what happens."

"How are we going to pay for it?"

"I don't know. If it's what we are supposed to do, the money will show up. After all, $5,000-plus per month, we don't have that kind of money. We don't even make that much in a month. If the money comes, we'll know what we're supposed to do," I reasoned.

"Yeah, well, it'll take a miracle to come up with $14,000 by next week, so don't get your hopes up."

A couple of days after our return from Houston, Mom came over to visit. Robby was lying around watching Ricky play, as he had done daily since his discharge from the hospital. Ricky went into his room, retrieving one of Robby's dinosaurs.

As Robby saw Ricky playing with his toy, he reached out his right arm and sound began to emerge from his lips. "Mmmmmmmmmmmmmiiiiiinnne (Mine)!" he yelled.

"Robby, you talked!" Rick, Mom, and I called out in unison.

My prayers were beginning to be answered, but I wanted more than healing for Robby. I wanted total restoration—for my son to be his old self, inside and out. Each day I prayed for every limb, every organ, and every cell to be as good as it had been before—or better. However long it took didn't matter. For the riches we sought were not hidden in faraway lands. They were right in front of us. If we could only see with the eyes of a child, we'd find them.

LESLIE GRAHAM

9

ADVENTURE

*The dusty overland trail was covered with signs of mass migration—
littered with debris from old food, livestock carcasses, even burial
sites of people unable to survive the expedition. From Missouri to
California, the half-mile-wide trail became home to thousands of
settlers for their six-month journey west. Covered wagons pulled by
oxen and mules were followed closely by those traveling on foot.
Tempted by the news of gold, entire families risked the challenges
with weather, cholera, and Indians for the limitless opportunity. The
potential to find abundant wealth captivated people's imaginations
and spurred these "49ers" westward.*

*Gold was found many times in centuries past, but never had
there been a gold rush. This was because, historically, a king,
emperor, or czar owned rights to all the gold found on their lands.
This time, however, in the land of liberty, the gold was free for the
taking.*

*During this time, a well-known phrase became popular
among nearly all California gold seekers. It was based on a story
about a farmer who risked all he had to visit a circus for the thrill of
seeing an elephant—something he wished for his entire life but had
never done. Though he lost all that he risked, he was so thrilled to
see the elephant that he didn't care about his losses, saying, "I don't
give a hang, for I have seen the elephant."[1]*

For 49ers, the elephant symbolized "suffering a severe ordeal, facing one's worst expectations, overcoming the meanest realities."[2] "Seeing the elephant" became a catchphrase for the experience that "like the farmer's circus elephant, was an exotic sight and unequaled experience, the adventure of a lifetime."[3]

"I talked to Mike today," Rick said.

"About what?" I asked.

"Do you remember the car wash he told us about?"

Before our trip to North Carolina, the firemen had begun planning an event to raise money for Robby. I hadn't forgotten, but I was easily distracted by the demands of the other parts of my life. I had resumed working full time, and Rick was back to work too. He stayed home with the kids on the days I worked and vice versa. We were all doing our best to be happy, pretending for a little while that we were normal again.

"Yes. What about it?" I asked.

"Well, he says they're getting a larger response from the community than they expected."

"That's great!"

"We're going down to the radio station in the morning to be on Mason & Nancy's morning show." Rick smiled, clearly happy at the prospect.

"You're kidding."

"I don't know how they got involved, but the station manager is really excited and wants to do something to help. At least we can get some free publicity for the car wash coming up."

I wished I could go, but I had to work. "I'll be sure to have my radio tuned in."

"Oh, another thing, they want us to make an appearance at the car wash, if Robby's feeling up to it. I guess a lot of people want to see him in person."

"Really? Why?" I asked.

"I don't know, but I'm not sure he's strong enough to be out there for very long."

"Rick, they're putting a lot of effort into this. I think we should try to show up, at least for a little while." How long could it take to make an appearance at a car wash?

Saturday, June 29, 1996

It was a perfect day for an outdoor fund-raiser. The clear sky and shining sun gave no indication of the forecasted rain. Though we needed it badly, I selfishly prayed for God to keep the rain away. Returning Robby to Houston required a lot of money. We needed all the help we could get, including the sun.

Of course, we needed more than good weather. Hopefully the firemen's trip to the radio station would pay off and bring lots of people to the car wash.

We loaded the kids in the van and headed to the event, wanting to get there early in the day so Robby could stay as long as possible before the immense summer heat kicked in.

"Hey Mike, we're on our way. What? I can't hear you," Rick spoke loudly into the big brick phone. "Wow, it's really noisy there. Oh yeah? Really?" He set the phone on his shoulder a second to whisper to me. "You're not going to believe this."

"You're kidding me!" He chuckled, listening to Mike again. The huge smile on his face indicated some measure of success. "Okay. We're right around the corner. We'll see you in a minute."

"You are *not* going to believe this," he said again to all of us.

Robby was ready to bounce out of his car seat, excited about the big party the firemen were having for him.

Rick continued, "Mike said there are so many people there, they can't begin to count them all. He just kept shouting, 'Wait 'til you see this!' "

As he described their conversation, we rounded the corner to our final destination. The traffic was much heavier than usual for a Saturday morning.

Robby began shouting, "My parade! My parade!" It was the best way he could understand what was happening.

As the corner came into view, we couldn't believe our eyes. The event spread over two parking lots covering adjacent corners of a busy six-lane intersection. Several sheriff's deputies directed traffic, intermittently stopping the flow of cars to allow people to cross the street.

An aerial fire truck with the ladder extended led the event on one corner. A dozen or more firefighters, in assembly line fashion, used long-handled brushes to clean the endless stream of cars, all awaiting the unique opportunity to have their vehicle washed with a fire hose.

On the opposite corner, a wide range of activities were offered. There was a dunking booth, a miniature fire truck giving rides, and remote-control police cars. The aroma of hotdogs, hamburgers, popcorn, and other delicious foods filled the air. Antique fire trucks were on display, as were modern fire trucks and equipment from nearby cities and districts. Firefighter demonstrations took place on a tower erected for the event. This and more inspired people to stuff dollar bills of every denomination into donation buckets all day long.

A multitude of companies held raffles for donated prizes. Pictures of Robby were on display at every booth. The radio station was broadcasting live from the event, and the sheriff's department was there for security. Helicopters from area hospitals also dropped in intermittently for brief exhibits. People swarmed these large birds for the rare opportunity to take a look inside.

The turnout was awesome. People were everywhere! With all of the media coverage, Robby had become somewhat of a local celebrity. All day, people shared their well wishes, prayers, and love with us. Midday, a black-haired gentleman in a deputy's uniform approached us.

"Hello, Mr. and Mrs. Graham." He introduced himself, looked down at the ground, then back at us hesitantly. "Would you mind if I say a little prayer for Robby?" he asked.

Rick and I looked at each other, smiling. "Sure," I answered.

The deputy reached into his shirt pocket and lifted out a small vial of clear liquid. He motioned us in closer, not wanting anyone else to view his tiny treasure. "I hope you don't think this is too weird, but I'd like to bless him with this."

"O . . . k . . . ay," Rick answered somewhat hesitantly, his face covered with questions.

The officer went on. "You see . . . I don't really know how to explain this . . . but . . . I just know I was supposed to bring this here today."

His response left our questions unanswered. Our facial expressions urged him to continue.

"You see, I was at a prayer meeting at church a couple of nights ago when a couple came in, home from a trip to Lourdes."

I gasped. My eyes widened.

"You've heard of it?" he asked.

I nodded my head yes. "I watched *The Song of Bernadette* only a few days ago."

Rick looked at us quizzically, not knowing to what the officer and I were referring.

I explained further, "There is this spring in France that is believed to have healing powers. The movie was about how it was discovered. It's a long story. Anyway . . . people come from all over the world to get in that water. Many claim to have been healed there."

The officer continued his story. "That's right. So this couple brought two vials of that water with them to the prayer meeting, knowing someone would be there who needed it."

"Wow, that's incredible," Rick replied.

"Once people knew what this couple had, they started to crowd in, begging for one of the vials. I was standing in the back, against the wall. There were so many others who needed it more than I did. "

"So how did you end up with a vial?" I asked.

"The man walked back to me, handed me a vial, and said, 'Here, you need this.' I didn't know what for until I found out I was going to be working this event."

When I'd watched that movie, I wished I could get Robby to Lourdes, France. I would've done anything to bring him to that pool. Now God was bringing the pool to us.

The three of us huddled together as the officer led a prayer for Robby's healing. His index finger, moistened with the precious water, drew the sign of the cross on Robby's forehead. As he prayed, the eyes of this strapping, authoritative man began to tear. His outer appearance was rock-solid strength, but inside he was soft clay, willing to mold lovingly to a sensitive situation for people he didn't even know. In admiration, I witnessed God's touch on the heart of this mighty man as he became emotional about our little boy. Though this officer was there to comfort us, I found myself wanting to comfort him. The strong force inside my heart assured me we were going to be fine.

As the day continued, I was amazed—not only at the turnout but at the supportive spirit of so many. Numerous people sacrificed a great amount of time and energy toward the success of this event. For weeks they were on phones, sending faxes, and going door-to-door to local businesses requesting donations. Every piece of equipment, the prizes, and all the food and drink were donated.

Near the end of the day, Mike came out of the sheriff's motor home to check on us. "We just did a count on the money so far and it looks pretty good," he reported.

"Yeah? How close are we?" Rick asked.

"Pretty close," Mike answered. "I think we're going to get enough for you to take Robby back to Dr. Burzynski."

"You've made that much?" I asked. "In one day?"

"We've got about three or four thousand dollars to go, but we haven't counted the call-in donations to the radio station yet."

Mike was an amazing blessing. He knew that even with two insurance policies, many expenses wouldn't be covered and our costs would mount. He was an answer to prayer, a special blessing sent from above, and a brilliant light that shined brightly in our darkest hours. He put everything he had into this event. It was a great turnout, but would it be enough?

A few hours later, the count was finally in. With the car wash, phone-in donations to the radio station, and donations by mail, the Robby Graham Cancer Fund now contained just over $14,000. We were going to Houston!

Our airfare was covered via tickets donated from a major airline, and with help from a nonprofit organization, our room and board for the trip were also paid. The treatment would cost another five thousand dollars per month, for approximately nine to twelve months. We didn't know how, but were sure that the Lord would provide that as well.

We knew we had to tell the doctors our decision eventually, but for now we wanted to keep it to ourselves. Then, a few days before our scheduled trip, the phone rang.

"Hello," I answered.

"Hello, Mrs. Graham, this is Dr. Friedman from Duke," the voice on the other end informed me.

I winced. "Hi, Henry," I chimed back, trying to hide my real feelings with sweetness in my voice.

"We are ready to get things started here for Robby. I'm calling to find out what you've decided."

I knew that he expected us to choose his facility. Perhaps, even our local hospital. It was clear from our last conversation that the Burzynski Clinic was not on our list of options, as far as he was concerned. I didn't know how to tell him.

"Well . . . I think we're going to try the Antineoplastons," I told him.

"You can't be serious. Do you have any idea what kind of risk you're taking with your son?"

"I think so."

"Mrs. Graham, medulloblastoma is very serious. A recurrence means certain death. You don't have time to play games."

"I understand what you're saying, but we don't want to cause him more harm. He's already in frail health since the surgery."

"I can't believe you are really considering going through with this. Do you realize that in six weeks' time you could be right back where you started?" he drilled.

I recalled the stark reality of the statistic that was regularly thrown at us. The recent memories of each doctor's opinion assaulted my mind while Henry continued pressuring me.

"Chemo and radiation are the only chance he has. These are the treatments recommended by every major medical center in the country."

"I realize that, but—"

"Mrs. Graham . . . if you don't do what we are recommending, I guarantee you your son will be dead within a year."

I was shocked. How was I supposed to answer that? My mind tried to process the blunt delivery of his prediction. Eventually Henry broke the uncomfortably long silence.

"Well . . . sometimes miracles happen," he conceded.

A huge smile spread across my face. "Yes, Henry, sometimes miracles *do* happen," I responded, followed by a pause of brief silence. "I tell you what. Let me talk to my husband and I'll get back to you," I told him, knowing full well that our minds would not be changed. We said our good-byes and I hung up the phone, relieved that the call was over.

We opened the door to the tiny space that would be our Houston home for the coming weeks. The two-room unit housed a tiny bathroom with room for tub and toilet alone. The sink and vanity were out in the main room, which had space enough for a king-size bed and television. Next to the bed was a tiny table with two chairs.

A strict budget, and stricter diet, ruled out eating in restaurants as much as possible. With a Styrofoam cooler as our refrigerator and the remaining groceries in a brown paper sack in the corner, our makeshift kitchen was stocked.

Before leaving home, we'd employed a nutritionist, who placed us on a dietary regimen much different than our usual meals. It consisted mostly of vegetables, some fruit, small portions of chicken and fish, no artificial flavors or colors, and *no* sugar or sugar substitutes. It was difficult to stick to while living on the road, but a couple of weeks on it had already relieved Robby from all medication, and every symptom of asthma had disappeared, making the dietary sacrifices worth continuing.

Due to a miscommunication, however, we were unable to start treatment as soon as we arrived. Apparently we needed to attend training classes, and Robby couldn't be placed on therapy until we were trained on the equipment. We spent a few days at the hotel waiting to start the training. Ricky and Amanda were home with my sister. I missed them so much, but at the same time, it was a relief to not have to worry about taking care of them on this trip too.

Once trained on how to run the pump and administer the medication, we spent entire days at the clinic. There were daily blood tests, more training, monitoring of weights and vital signs, and checkups by the doctors.

The third day of Robby's treatment, we decided to take in a movie. It was Fourth of July weekend, and a movie would help us escape the blistering heat and deliver us from reality for a few hours. Though we arrived at the mall with time to spare, the lines at the theater were long, so we decided to go to the vitamin store before purchasing our movie tickets. Rick wheeled Robby through the narrow aisles of GNC. Suddenly Robby began vomiting.

I leaned in, stroking his little face. "Oh baby, are you okay?" I asked.

He nodded yes, but his eyes said otherwise.

"Come on, we've got to go," Rick urged.

An awkward struggle between fear and embarrassment took over my insides.

"What about—"

Rick was already pushing the wheelchair toward the exit. "We're really sorry," he called to a store employee as we rushed out.

He took Robby to the men's room to clean up. There would be no movie.

I waited outside. *Oh no*, I thought, my insides started to twist. *Vomiting with headaches is a symptom of increasing pressure in the brain. I hope he isn't already getting worse again. Did we make the wrong choice?*

We returned to the hotel and called the clinic. They sent over IV fluids and told us to take him off the medication until Monday. I agreed, though I wanted him to stay on the treatment. This was all taking much longer to get under way than I wanted.

On Monday we returned to the clinic expecting another long day, as usual. Rick was in his Grinch-like mood, but Robby was feeling better and showing signs of increased energy. Eventually we were in a room with Dr. Burzynski and Dr. Rita.

"We have found that his uric acid levels are high. They have increased quite a bit since starting treatment," Dr. Burzynski reported.

"What does that mean?" Rick asked. "Is that bad?"

"Well, it can be bad if levels get too high, but this is effect of tumor breakdown."

"His tumor is breaking down?"

"Yes."

"How do you know that?" Rick asked in a stern voice.

"Increased uric acid levels coincide with tumor breakdown. We usually see this between day 3 and 5 on treatment. So it is good sign that treatment is working," Dr. B answered.

"You mean to tell me you have a medicine that can start to break down his tumor in just three days!?" Rick yelled.

They nodded their heads and smiled.

I didn't know what to think. Either these people were some of the best liars I had ever met, or they were very sincere people who were being persecuted by the medical establishment.

"I am quite happy with results so far, but we will need to reduce medication."

"Why?" I asked. I wanted them to keep going if it was working so well.

"Well, this is making him sick, and we can achieve same result at lower dosage, only slower."

What a relief. Robby wasn't getting worse—he was getting better.

After two weeks, it was time for me to return home. I had to get back to work again, and Amanda and Ricky needed to be home too. Rick and Robby would follow me in a week or so, as soon as Dr. B felt Robby was stable enough to be monitored long distance.

Back at home, I waited eagerly for Rick to call and say they were coming home. I was at work when he finally called.

"Leslie, your husband is on line 2," a nurse told me.

My heart raced. *Why is he calling me at work?* I tried to stay calm. "Hello?"

"Hi," he replied abruptly.

"What's the matter?" I asked.

"Well, they're ready to discharge us, but Dr. Solomon won't sign the papers."

"What do you mean?"

"The people in the office here said that they can't let us go home until a local doctor signs the papers to be a co-investigator."

"But Dr. Solomon told us he didn't have any problem with that."

"Yeah, well, I guess he changed his mind. They said his secretary told them that he read the paperwork and he's not going to sign it."

"I don't understand. We talked to him about this before we went to Texas. He said that he would sign the FDA papers so Robby could be in the trial."

"I don't know. I've called them over and over again. I don't know what kind of game they're playing, but I'm tired of this crap. I can't get through to him. Can you try? I want to get out of this flippin' place."

"Sure. I'll call right now."

I hung up the phone and instantly dialed Dr. Solomon's office.

"Pediatric Neurosurgery, how can I help you?" the receptionist answered.

"Hello, this is Mrs. Graham. My son Robby is a patient of Dr. Solomon's."

"Yes."

"Can I talk with the doctor?"

"No, you may not," she answered rudely.

"Why not?"

"Mrs. Graham, Dr. Solomon is not going to sign those papers and he's *not* going to talk to you about it."

"Why? He told us that he would sign them."

"Well, he's not going to."

I wanted to know why! Why didn't he tell us that from the beginning? This was our first lesson in the politics of medicine. I couldn't believe what I was hearing. Now what would we do? I didn't want to relocate to Texas. What would Rick and I do for a living? We were both licensed to work in Florida. It would take time to get licensed to work in another state. I didn't want my family to have to live apart either.

I called Rick back. "Of course the receptionist wouldn't let me talk to Dr. Solomon," I told him. "And she was certainly ready for my call. She was quite rude and told me that he absolutely refused to sign those papers."

"Did you find out why?" he asked.

"No." We were both silent for a moment. "What do we do now?"

"They just told me that we have to find a doctor," Rick replied.

"Let me try Dr. White."

I hung up and dialed our pediatrician's office to request an immediate appointment. The doctors at the hospital had expressed their lack of confidence, in a condescending way, whenever they talked about good old Dr. White. He was pretty laid back, an old-fashioned kind of doc. He didn't rush patients through like cattle and even had a $350 annual limit that families paid out-of-pocket per year. I've never seen another doctor do that since. Fortunately, his receptionist let me come in to meet with the doctor that same afternoon.

Soon I was sitting in one of his exam rooms waiting to talk to him in person. "Hello, Mrs. Graham. What can I do for you today?" Dr. White pulled up his stool to sit next to me.

"My husband is in Houston right now with Robby. We got him into a clinical trial for a special medication that doesn't have all of the complications and side effects of traditional chemo."

"That sounds very interesting."

"Dr. Solomon originally agreed to sign the FDA papers as co-investigator to monitor Robby locally, but now he's changed his mind for some reason and they can't come home until we get those papers signed."

"Well, I have a letter here from the hematology-oncology doctors."

Dr. White pulled a paper from Robby's chart and proceeded to read the letter to me. It told him how bad Dr. B's treatment was and what a huge mistake it was for us to make this decision against their advice. It demanded that he stick together with them and refuse to cooperate with us. I was devastated.

Talk about an underhanded move. This was now a conspiracy. Our own doctors were secretly discussing and planning our failure on Burzynski's treatment. They were trying to stop us even before we could get started. How dare they try to influence another doctor and not tell us? It was as if this group of doctors got together and collectively thought of ways to keep us off the treatment. They had to know that we would need a local doctor and that our pediatrician was the logical choice. They covered that base by writing to him, trying to get him on their side. Now what were we going to do?

"I'll do it," Dr. White said decisively.

Wow. Did I hear him right?

As his pen touched down on the paper, my eyes confirmed what my ears still doubted; ink flowed from the pen as it moved across the page. I was pleasantly amazed. At least there was still one doctor willing to do the right thing. He signed the papers and they were faxed to Dr. B's clinic that afternoon.

Rick and Robby were coming home! I wasn't sure how Rick would feel about the television cameras at the airport. Living in the public eye was beginning to wear on us already, but it was necessary in order to maintain support for Robby. All of the publicity was a good thing. Lack of money was no longer our challenge, and Robby's treatment was well on course, but our adventure had just begun.

Like the 49ers, we were on a journey to find treasure—not gold or silver but riches that money can't buy. Hassle or not, it was all worth it, for we were going to see the elephant!

10
FACT VS. TRUTH

A multitude of hooves galloped across eleventh-century Europe. The gallant cloud of noblemen, red crosses emblazoned proudly across their chests, courageously marched on to their final destiny. As their noble steeds trampled across the sandy desert lands, trumpets blared and a Holy War began. Thousands gave their lives for the cause; their sacrifice, an act of honor. With quivers full and hearts impassioned, they pressed on, committed to bringing truth to the Middle East—their goal, to reclaim the Holy Land.

For nearly two centuries, the battles continued. In time, the mission of truth became plagued by greed. Horrific brutality ensued. Those who once vowed to "stop the infidel" now spread carnage throughout an entire continent. Mass executions of civilians prevailed—terrorizing Muslims, Christians, and Jews. Yet to this day, Western and Eastern perspectives of the facts surrounding the Crusades vary greatly. Which facts are true?

This thing called truth is a subject of great debate. Simple enough for the common man to follow, yet it forges complex discussion among the minds of the elite. It has inspired men both great and small on massive quests. Some find it easily. Though, even after the deepest search, it escapes others. Now I was on my own crusade to locate it.

All the doctors on Robby's case performed within their own view of the facts, each in perfect alignment with their own opinion of reality. Yet they varied greatly from one another. Were they all revealing fact or truth?

Disagreeing opinions on whose facts are true often result in conflict, even among the most educated, intelligent of professionals. Our experience would be no different.

It had been nearly two months since we'd seen Dr. Solomon. I was supportive of my husband, who was still angry with him for not signing the FDA papers, but I was nervous about this appointment. I feared my own wounds were too newly healed and might reopen when I saw him, but I needed to trust this doctor. Moreover, I believed in time his decision would prove to be in error, and I wanted to be there when he realized it.

When Dr. Solomon walked in, he was totally business. Perhaps he too had preconceived notions of our reaction and wanted to remain distant.

This isn't so bad, I thought as he examined Robby.

Suddenly Robby looked intently at Dr. Solomon, eye to eye, with a very stern look and asked, "Why didn't you sign my papers?"

Rick looked at me with wide eyes, and I at him.

Dr. Solomon replied, "What did you say?" as though he didn't understand what Robby was talking about.

I turned my head to hide the smile on my face, trying hard not to laugh. I was so surprised. I hadn't realized that Robby was even aware of the situation, but he'd obviously paid attention. Maybe I should've expected it. He regularly instructed the nurses as to whether they were drawing his labs incorrectly or changing his needles wrong. He watched *everything*.

Dr. Solomon played it cool and didn't really give Robby an answer. Rick and I smiled, allowing the man to stew in his own juices. He had to know exactly what Robby was talking about, but we pretended right along with him. That was fine with me. Dr. Solomon was the only doctor for several hundred miles who could perform this type of surgery, if Robby needed it, and I didn't want anyone else. I still liked him. He was an outstanding surgeon, in spite of our disagreement on treatment.

"Well, let me put up the recent scan," he said, placing the films from Robby's most current MRI up on the screen for us to see.

We weren't sure what to expect, but the miserable feeling that accompanied our initial visit to the emergency room was missing.

"I'm very pleased with these films," he announced.

The MRI report indicated no abnormal enhancement. This was an improvement. There remained, however, an area of concern that was thought to be metastatic nodules in Robby's left ventricle. This hadn't changed. Although we would've preferred for it to disappear, it wasn't enhanced and hadn't grown. At least there was no progression of disease. The fact that there were no longer areas of enhancement was an improvement. Dr. Burzynski's treatment was working!

After informing us of the good news, Dr. Solomon requested, "Tell me more about what you're doing."

He seemed sincerely interested in the protocol for Burzynski's Antineoplaston therapy. So we abandoned our oath to ourselves, having planned to shelter the local doctors from information about Robby's new treatment for fear they'd use it to work against us again. However, the protocol was specified by the FDA and available to the public; it was no secret. In light of Robby's positive results, I enthusiastically explained the details to Dr. Solomon, who appeared to receive them with great interest and hope.

We were ecstatic about the recent turn of events. Robby was getting better, and it seemed we had a renewed ally in Dr. Solomon. Leaving his office that day, down the long corridor to the elevators, Rick, Robby, and I ran, holding hands and giggling all the way.

The next month or so was uneventful, with August nearly over. The Burzynski Patient Group, initially started by a few extremely determined individuals, was hard at work to save from persecution the doctor who so graciously worked tirelessly to save their lives. We began receiving their mailings with increased frequency after beginning treatment, and this recent flyer indicated another hurdle on our path to healing:

RALLY TO SUPPORT CANCER PATIENTS

Demonstrate in support of every American's right to freely choose the medical treatment of their choice

WHEN: Saturday, September 28, 1996 – Noon to 3 p.m.
WHERE: Pennsylvania Ave. in front of White House
Washington, D.C.

Robby's overall health was improving and life was beginning to approach the ordinary. While still getting acclimated to our new "normal," we were beginning to learn more about the intimate details of Dr. Burzynski's legal troubles. The issues we so easily ignored on our initial visit began to loom larger as they now affected us personally.

Though we were doing well on one hand, the very thing helping us do so well was now being threatened. Robby was currently enrolled in an FDA-approved clinical trial, but only six months earlier, Dr. Burzynski's office was raided by FBI agents who held patients captive while they removed file cabinets loaded with patient information. Many things had occurred in the six months since; most were beneficial to Dr. B and his beloved patients. The FDA had officially approved sixty-eight clinical trials, yet still they were on a mission to prosecute our doctor for the crime of treating patients who had crossed state lines to be treated. The FDA calls this "interstate commerce of an unapproved drug."

Amongst the fund-raisers and doctor visits to save Robby's life, we were now battling to save his doctor too.

The account that the firemen had established funded all of Robby's medical expenses (that weren't covered by insurance), and generous companies and individuals filled in the gaps, paying for all of Robby's treatment-related travel expenditures. Expenses for defending his doctor, however, were going to fall squarely upon us.

I was fortunate to still have my job, but costs were mounting and so was our debt. No matter. Fueled with determination in my spirit and passion in my heart, I would get to that rally one way or another.

While I flew into Washington D.C. with Rick's mom, Sharron, and his brother Darren, Rick and Robby were en route to Houston for Robby's first checkup with Dr. B. Completing a series of plane, bus, and train rides, we emerged from Union Station. My heart fluttered and I stood tall as my eyes set upon a view of the U.S. Capitol across the street. Reminded of those who had gone before me, the monument to patriotism was a symbol of all who were willing to fight for freedom. I felt a surge of gratitude and strength, mixed with a sense of destiny, at the opportunity to come to this place with the freedom to make my voice heard.

After walking several blocks through the historic streets, we arrived at our hotel. From our window we could see the hoopla surrounding a Clinton fund-raising dinner at the hotel across the street. We went downstairs for a closer look, watching from the sidewalk.

"There he is! There he is!" Sharron shouted while slapping me repeatedly on my right shoulder.

As she excitedly grabbed my attention, I scanned the crowded driveway looking for the man that captured her interest. Senator Ted Kennedy was emerging from a limo.

Having spent half of her life in Massachusetts, the senator was a big deal to her. She was star struck. "This is so amazing."

Limousines carrying congressmen, senators, and other dignitaries lined the driveway of this grand hotel.

I didn't share her enthusiasm. While my son fought for his life and his doctor fought for his freedom, these people who could make a difference were busy having parties for thousands of dollars per plate.

In the days that followed, we spent every waking hour lobbying with senators and congressmen. Before spanning out across Washington D.C., the Burzynski Patient Group held a meeting with our lobbyist, Tony Martinez. The leadership of our group had hired him to represent patients and families, giving us a voice and presence in Washington beyond our current visit. He had already been working on our behalf for months.

Being a lobbyist, he knew the intricacies of dealing with congressional representatives and wanted to send us out armed with correct information, prepared to speak on our own behalf intelligently. The room filled with people. Although some of the patients and family members had testified in support of Dr. B at congressional hearings a few months earlier, the vast majority of us were new to this terrain.

Tony informed us, "Remember, when you are talking with these congressmen and senators, you are trying to get them to do something for which no legal precedence has been set. You have no right to medical freedom."

Faces around the room were stunned into silence as we all tried to process what we just heard.

How can I, an American citizen, have no right to say what I do or do not want done to my body? I wondered. I couldn't believe it. I had never heard anything like this.

I raised my hand, "What about the right to life, liberty, and the pursuit of happiness?"

"Yes, you may have the right to life, liberty, and the pursuit of happiness," Tony answered, "but no right to medical freedom. Nowhere does the constitution state that you have a right to choose medical treatment for your body. There is no law that gives you that right."

An angry mumble of disagreement quietly roared through the room.

Why do I need a law for that? I thought. *This is craziness.* I felt like a kid who just discovered that magic isn't real. I had lazily floated through life simply accepting as truth all the great things I had been taught in school about freedom and choice in America. And now—the curtain was pulled and the deceitful tricks revealed. Had things really progressed in this country to a place where only the government could say what was right and wrong for my body and my health?

More questions by others in the group followed, all of us progressively angrier as the answers continued to clarify the mountain that lie before us. I had no idea how strongly politics and medicine were entwined, and I was certain that most Americans had no clue how limited their rights to medical freedom really were. My fury gave way to a renewed energy to talk to as many legislators as possible during our short stay.

From there, each of us spent the next two days with our own congressional representatives, periodically meeting together as a group. Senator Connie Mack was our representative from Florida. He had recently had his own bout with cancer. Surely he would be sympathetic to our cause. When we got to his office, I was disappointed that we had to meet with an aide. The senator did not have time to meet with us himself.

Later though, Sharron and Darren were fortunate to meet personally with Florida Congressman Bill Young, while I went with a group of parents to meet with Congressman Jim Moran. Unfortunately he was not available at the time either.

Eventually, in some of the large group meetings, we were able to meet with congressional representatives Joe Barton, Richard Burr, and Peter DeFazio.

The three-day trip ended with the rally to which the flyer had originally beckoned us. It was a chilly fall day with the sun hiding behind low, grey clouds—not a spot of sunlight. Near the White House, in Lafayette Park, a small stage had been erected, surrounded by a multitude of Burzynski supporters.

The gloomy, overcast day did little to help me fight the many emotions swirling inside. I wanted to believe everything was going to be alright. It had been an exciting week filled with moments of empowerment. Meeting with influential men in Congress was an experience that I would've never dreamed I'd have. How exciting to have the ear of the many someones who have the ability to change the laws! All were sympathetic to our cause. They said they understood and would help us fight, yet thoughts and feelings stirring inside me caused me to wonder whether that would ever really happen.

Standing, waiting for the rally to begin, I thought about Rick and Robby. *I wonder what they're doing right now*, I thought to myself. *I sure wish they were here.* I knew they would have loved to participate, but Robby's appointment with Dr. B was just as important. As my mind wrapped in thoughts of my family, my gaze wandered around the park.

Princess Diana, who was visiting the White House, was strolling in the background, followed by a cluster of men, presumably bodyguards.

Oh, it would be so wonderful if she would join our cause, I wishfully thought to myself. We had some celebrity support—Larry Gatlin was an advocate—but we needed more. To me, if we could only get enough of the right support, word would soon get out and this battle could be easily won. As the news cameras lined up, I was hopeful that somehow we'd get enough attention to turn things around.

The rally was kicked off by Steve Siegel. He and his wife, Mary Jo, founded the Burzynski Patient Group. She was a patient and strong supporter of Dr. B.

"One year after starting Dr. Burzynski's treatment," Mary Jo spoke, "UCLA announced me in remission. Dr. Burzynski saved my life, and for that he is facing three hundred years in a federal penitentiary."

Congressman Frank Pallone gave a great speech in support of Dr. Burzynski and his patients. Tom Wilbanks, head of the Texas chapter of Citizens for Health, also gave an inspiring speech, raising awareness of the many groups fighting for our right to health freedom. The crowd cheered each speaker, applauding and waving their signs in the air.

Mrs. Burzynski, back from a recent trip to Rome, spoke as well. Only a few days prior, the *Washington Times* reported, "Cancer doctor sees pope, but not about his health."[1] Dr. Burzynski and his wife, Barbara, were summoned by the pontiff, who wanted to learn more about Dr. B's research. He personally prayed blessing upon them for success in their battle with the FDA.

She proudly announced, "One day the world will know that this great man fought for what he believes, and the world will have a cure for cancer!"

As cameras from local and national media rolled, the patients and their families eventually had a turn to speak.

One mom emotionally reported, "If it wasn't for Dr. Burzynski, our son would be dead." Her now-healthy fifteen-year-old son stood at her side.

A precious eight-year-old patient stepped to the microphone, and in his sweet little voice told the crowd, "If it wasn't for Dr. Burzynski, I wouldn't be here."

"Why is the government doing this?" cried another. "It's not fair!" Tears formed in my eyes as I listened to this woman's pleas. *It isn't fair. Why don't they just leave us alone?*

The resistance coming from the government was masked as protection. Yet here were the ones the FDA was claiming to protect—the very ones who were fighting hard to get the government out of their way so they could get treatment.

Over and over patients stepped to the microphone.

"They have no right to tell us what we can do to our bodies," yelled one.

We have something that works. Why can't we be left in peace? We just want to live! I thought.

Another patient said, "The FDA has made a list and has decided who can live and who will die."

Cheers roared on in unison with waving signs. As the procession of speakers continued to step up to the mic, the crowd grew in both size and volume. The rising level of anger coming from the masses drove hearts and minds to united resolution—kicking my own obstinate determination into high gear.

After the rally, the protest moved as we marched along the well-manicured lawn of the White House, chanting, "FDA . . . go away . . . let us live another day!"

Free Dr. B
Save the Doctor Who Saves Lives!
Dr. Burzynski Patient Group

The large blue banner led the sea of white signs that were bouncing up and down as our chanting continued. Among them: "Save the Doctor Who Is a Life Saver," "Living Proof," "Help Us Win the War on Cancer," "Right to Choose, Right to Live," "FDA Is Playing God with Our Lives," and many more.

Near the front of the entourage, a sign displaying a poster-sized photo of Robby waved high among the ocean of signs. On it, large black letters boldly cried out, "Don't Let Me Die." I carried my sign proudly, chanting with the rest of the voices, hoping to bring attention to our plight. Sharron and Darren carried similar signs right alongside me.

While protesting, I couldn't help but wonder, *How on earth did this happen? My life wasn't supposed to turn out this way. I should be home living a normal life not angrily screaming against the FDA in our nation's capital,* I thought to myself as we marched along. I feared the worst and hoped for the best all while wishing this nightmare had never begun.

Being a demonstrator for any cause was never an aspiration of mine. Campaigns against government conspiracies were for left-winged radicals, not normal people like me. At least that's what I had always believed. Never could I have imagined that I would be picketing in front of the White House for a chance to save my child's life.

When it was all said and done, over 175 present and former patients, their families, and other supporters of Dr. Burzynski were in attendance, firmly banded together to save the lives of Dr. B and his patients.

The days spent in Washington proved to be fruitful to some extent. Hundreds of supporters made personal contacts with their elected officials, and it looked as though we made an impression. Many congressmen were now taking an active interest in our plight. Though I did not have a chance to attend meetings with them, others in Washington who supported us were Senators Orrin Hatch and Tom Daschle, and Representatives Frank Pallone, Dan Frisa, Jim Moran, J. D. Hayworth, and Tom Harkin. We were grateful to these honorable men for their support.

But . . . would that support be enough?

I wondered.

Though we had gained support in Congress, the trial started as scheduled. On January 6, 1997, we were back in Houston for the first in a series of hearings related to Dr. Burzynski's trial. Over three months had passed since our visit to Washington D.C., and it seemed we still had support coming from our elected officials. We received a copy of the following letter, dated January 3, 1997:

> To the Patients of Dr. Stanislaw Burzynski and their families:
> I would like to take this opportunity to reassure you that the Congress will do everything we can to see to it that your access to Antineoplaston therapy continues as prescribed by your physician and the law.
> I know you and your families are concerned about the future. While I am unable to comment on Dr. Burzynski's trial, I do want to let you know that the Congress will continue monitoring this case closely. Whatever the outcome, my colleagues and I want your concerns as cancer patients to be properly addressed by the Food and Drug Administration (FDA). Please stay in touch with us and with your respective Representatives and Senators. Our thoughts and prayers are with you.
>
> Sincerely,
>
> Peter DeFazio
> Member of Congress[2]

Now in Texas, many of the same signs that graced the sidewalks of Washington D.C. paved the snow-dusted walkway in front of the federal courthouse in Houston.

"Save the doctor that's saving lives!" the protesters cried out in unison, their frosty breath visible in the air.

Dozens of cameras from news agencies all over the globe flashed repeatedly as patients took turns in front of the lectern to tell their stories and plead for common sense to prevail.

"You want to talk about a crime," Steve Siegel shouted at reporters, "look around you at all these people who should be busy trying to recover and fighting their cancer, but instead they have to be here in 35-degree weather, fighting for the right to their treatment. Ask yourself, why is this happening?"

Dawn Hall, whose husband, Tracy, was a patient, told journalists, "Put yourself in our shoes. It could be your spouse or your children."

Every patient wanted a chance to speak and make their case for freeing Dr. Burzynski, but only a limited number of us would be able to speak to the media.

Another woman stepped to the mic, "What he is doing is helping mankind."

I saw Mariann and Jack Kunnari there with Dustin. Robby and Dustin had become good friends, as had their parents. Rick and I made our way through the crowd to stand near them. Before I knew it, both Mariann and I found ourselves urged to the front. One thing our fellow supporters had learned from past events was that Mariann and I could be counted on for emotional pleas, and the sweet faces of our adorable, blond-haired little boys could melt even the hardest of hearts.

I watched Mariann go first and waited for my turn to speak. As I looked out upon the conglomerate of reporters and cameras, my heart began to race. I could feel beads of sweat forming under my coat while the numbness in my frozen fingers and toes throbbed.

Oh my gosh, I am going to be on national television. What am I going to say? Robby's MRI had been clean for six months, but he needed this treatment to stay that way. He still had a few more months left on the protocol, and I feared that without it, his cancer would return and . . . well . . . I didn't want to think about that.

My ears were half listening to the heartfelt words of Mariann, who began to cry as she begged for the nation to join us in our fight to free Dr. B—our best chance at a cure with a somewhat normal quality of life.

Tears began forming in my eyes. *I'm not going to cry. I'm not going to cry*, I repeated over and over to myself in concert with my racing heart.

Then it was my turn. I stepped to the microphone and Rick stood beside me with Robby in his arms. Looking out, the cameras seemed so close. My heart pounded even faster and I fought hard to keep the tears at bay. But all of the love, anger, fear—every emotion ever encountered on this journey—seemed to forge together inside me at one time. Combined with the cold winter air and the rapid beating of my heart, it took my breath away. Standing at the podium with tears streaming down my face, the flashing continued and the world looked on as I tried to gain my composure and speak.

"Please," I took a deep breath and in a shaky voice continued, "if Dr. Burzynksi is imprisoned and this treatment is taken away . . ." I paused to sniffle and then cried, "my son will die!"

The tears flowed and I couldn't speak anymore. A friend wrapped her arms around me and held me while I cried and Rick took over speaking.

I hated this. I hated all of it. I just wanted life to be normal again.

A while later, during a break from the trial, Dr. Burzynski stopped for a few minutes to talk too. "The truth is that this treatment works," he remarked. "It should be brought to the jury's attention."

That would never be. Whether the treatment worked or not wasn't important for the jury to know, the judge decided. Patients taking the medication over state lines—that's what mattered.

Every day patients gathered outside the federal courthouse. In the afternoons we would return to the clinic, line up on the leather sofas in Dr. B's waiting room, gather around the television, and watch the news, hoping for a glimpse of an end to all the madness.

Many times journalists and cameramen from various media accompanied us to the clinic. Angry patients were great interviews.

As much as we strived to communicate things accurately, the news people always had a twist—their view of the truth, I suppose. Before this, I never would've guessed how often that happened. But whether raising money for Robby or awareness for Dr. B, rarely were the facts reported as we gave them.

Among the reporters that we talked to was Charles Zewe from CNN, who reported, "When Robert and Leslie Graham's son had brain cancer, the outlook was grim. He was given a 20 percent chance to live. Today the cancer is gone; five-year-old Robbie's tumor is shrinking. And the federal government wants to put his doctor in jail."[3]

To clarify, my husband's name is Rick (not Robert), Robby
was given a 10 percent chance of surviving five years (0 percent if
we chose this treatment over conventional), and a tumor cannot be
simultaneously shrinking and gone. It was *gone*!

After a few days, we returned home and waited for news,
knowing that the trial would be lengthy. After four weeks the
prosecution finally rested. I was called to testify for the defense, so
in February we returned to Houston.

Again afternoons were spent at the courthouse. As we exited
for a lunch break, a reporter and her cameraman approached. "Can
you tell us about the trial going on inside?" she asked.

Rick pointed at me, "Ask her," he said smiling—ever the
prankster. He and Robby had been inside the courtroom for many
hours, and he knew I couldn't go in since I was a testifying witness.
Witnesses weren't allowed to go in for fear that their testimony
might be influenced by what we heard others say.

Instantly the microphone was at my lips and the camera in
my face. I raised my hand to keep the camera from touching my
skin. *Why do they have to get so close?* I wondered. "No comment,"
I answered.

"Don't you want people to know what's going on in there?"
she pressed.

"I'm a witness," I answered, my hand still raised in front of
the camera. "I haven't been inside yet, and I'm not supposed to
comment."

Of course I wanted people to know what kind of idiocy their
tax dollars were paying for, but I didn't want my testimony thrown
out because I talked to some reporter who in all likelihood would
report the facts wrong anyway. Honestly, I was tired of talking to
reporters. I just wanted to be left alone.

We spent the afternoons protesting, with more time in front
of cameras, and evenings meeting with attorneys. Sometimes we
would drive by the clinic at ten or eleven o'clock at night and see
Dr. Burzynski working in his office. I don't know how the man got
any sleep. He would go to the clinic early in the morning to review
patient charts and make recommendations. Then he would go to the
trial all day, come back in the afternoon to see patients, and work

late into the night completing all of the FDA-mandated paperwork for the clinical trials.

Back at the courthouse again, I and about a dozen other patients were summoned to stand by, waiting to be called to testify. I couldn't wait for the chance to bear witness. I only wished that I could tell them everything I thought, knew, and felt. But we were severely limited in what our testimony could include, unable to say anything in reference to the treatment working or patients being helped. I hoped that somehow, just the fact that I was an RN would register with the jury that this treatment wasn't snake oil and magic tricks. It was medicine that really worked.

"The defense calls Leslie Graham to the stand."

I stood and vowed to tell the truth, the whole truth, and nothing but the truth.

Dr. B's attorney asked, "Could you please state your name for the record?"

"Leslie Graham."

"And Mrs. Graham, what is your occupation?"

"I am a registered nurse."

"Are you a patient of Dr. Burzynski?"

"No, my five-year-old son is."

He asked a few more questions to clarify that the clinic did in fact conduct patient training, and then the prosecution had their turn, which they completed rather quickly.
I was on the stand less than five minutes. My brief testimony had me leaving the witness seat before it had time to warm. Clearly the prosecution didn't want a registered nurse representing their opposition.

The trial went on for two more weeks before going to jury. Finally, in March 1997, the deadlocked jury forced a mistrial. The judge acquitted Dr. Burzynski on thirty-four counts of mail fraud and set a new trial date of May 19 for the forty-one remaining charges. We were victorious for the time being, but the war was not yet finished.

There had been a number of facts in play during our crusade. Jaded by disappointments of the recent past, it became difficult to see a future without battles. After fighting one thing or another for nearly a year, combat was now a habit. We marched on, having learned to champion our own crusade. The fact is: Robby was doing well. We were onto something great. But facts can change. The truth, however, never changes.

11
TIME

It's been called the great equalizer. Through all of history it has been present, and how we decide to use it can make all the difference. Do we invest it or spend it? Do we utilize it or waste it? Failing to respect it can produce great loss, but harnessing its power will yield great abundance.

People often become content with the passing of it, comforted by a sense of security that frequently proves false.

Time. It's the one thing we all have the same amount of each day, but our control over it is limited. We can't slow it down or make it go faster. And as the busyness of our lives brings days rushing past, most of us wish we had more.

Ultimately we must release the timing of events to the only One who has authority to schedule the perfect moment—for all things have an appointed place in time.

Having spent twelve hours cramped in a rental car, I was actually happy to be back at Duke. Dr. Burzynski ordered a PET scan for Robby. At the time, Duke was one of the only places in our part of the country with one of these expensive machines.

Robby had been on treatment successfully for eight months, and we were preparing to complete the IV portion of the therapy. Yes!

PET scans detect metabolic activity of cells. Cancer cells have a higher metabolic rate than normal brain cells, so they gobble up the sugary serum, injected through a vein, and thus enhance on the scan. This is how abnormal growths, particularly those that might be too small to see on an MRI, could be detected. Robby also had an MRI taken just before we left home so that the radiologists could compare the two. I was a little sad to learn that our appointment was with Dr. Friedman's associate and not with Henry himself. I really wanted to see him eat all of the terrible words he proclaimed about Dr. Burzynski on our first visit. Not to mention that he was totally wrong about his guarantee that Robby would be dead within a year if we didn't follow his advice. The stuff worked— I couldn't wait for him to admit it. I had planned on taking great pleasure in telling him that I was right and he was wrong. Unfortunately I wouldn't be able to do so on this trip.

"It's just too bad we won't be able to see Henry's face when he finds out," I told Rick.

The scan was a simple procedure and didn't take long. Afterward we met with Dr. Longee back in Clinic.

"Robby appears to be doing very well," Dr. Longee said.

I smiled, "Yep, he sure is. I guess you guys were wrong about Dr. Burzynski."

"It could be, or it could just be anecdotal evidence. Dr. Burzynski refuses to submit to double-blind studies and appropriate scientific testing."

"Oh, come on," Rick urged, "who would volunteer for a double-blind study when they're dying of cancer? No one like that is going to submit to being the one to take a placebo. You guys don't even do that."

"Darrell, you know that's not true," I added. "Why don't you guys try it here?"

"Why would we offer something that's not proven when we have effective treatments available?"

"You know you don't have a cure, and the treatments you offer aren't that great," I countered. "They cause all kinds of horrific problems. Heck, some of them even cause secondary cancers."

"Yes, but they are the best we have right now, and we do get results for some people with them."

108

"So why don't you do a limited clinical trial with kids who have exhausted all traditional methods?"

"Because the political climate isn't conducive to working with Dr. Burzynski right now."

Well, there it was—the true reason. The fact is, pharmaceutical companies fund the research performed at the university level. Working with Dr. Burzynski could make the drug companies pull their financial backing. Then where would the university be? Better to turn their heads to something that worked than to upset the status quo. At least, that was my opinion. I wanted to rub their noses in it, but I realized they would never change course if we were too rude.

Rick asked, "So what about the scan we had today? When will we get the results?"

"You should get a copy of the report in about a week," Dr. Longee replied.

"Did you get a chance to look at the MRI scan we brought?" asked Rick.

"No, let's take a look at it now."

He placed the film up on the screen for all of us to see.

"Looks pretty good," he observed.

"What's that?" Rick asked, pointing at a small white spot in the cerebellar region.

"Oh my, I didn't see that. It's small, but it looks like there's a recurrence here."

In fact, there was an "8-millimeter enhancing nodule," the official MRI report would later read. All of my earlier excitement quickly deflated. How in the heck did this happen? Why did the treatment stop working?

"I'm really sorry, guys," Dr. Longee expressed sincerely.

"Well, I guess we'll have to see what Dr. Burzynski is going to do about this," I replied.

"Please keep us posted on the situation," Dr. Longee requested.

Regretfully I answered, "We will."

The long ride home was excruciatingly quiet. I could tell Rick was stunned and didn't want to talk. So I kept my thoughts to myself.

Out of the silence, Rick finally asked, "What do you think it is?"

"I don't know," I answered, staring out the window. I took a deep breath and blew it out slowly through pursed lips as the trees and bushes flashed by. "It looks like he has a recurrence."

"Damn it!" Rick yelled, pounding on the steering wheel.

I cringed closer to my window. "It'll be alright," I said, trying to calm him.

"No, it's not alright!"

"It's a tiny little dot. We don't even have an official report. Maybe it's nothing."

"It's *not* nothing!"

We drove on in silence for hours. Robby slept peacefully in the backseat while Rick and I retreated to our own imaginations.

Eventually Rick began talking again. "So . . . what's God telling you now?" he asked sarcastically.

"He hasn't told me anything."

"This really sucks."

"I have a really good feeling. I'm not worried about it."

"I am so damn sick of hearing you say that."

"What? That Robby's going to be fine? Well, I don't feel bad about it. It's all going to work out."

"What in the hell is the matter with you? Are you crazy? He has cancer in his head. You know what a recurrence means."

"I just don't believe it's over. God has everything under control."

"I sure hope you're right."

Maybe I am crazy, I thought, as our conversation ended. Yet I still had the same unexplainable feeling that everything would be okay.

Over the past months, multiple fund-raisers kept Robby's current treatment plan alive, but now the fund was running out of money. Maybe our time with this treatment was done. Before we had to make that decision, however, we learned that another large fund-raiser was in the works.

Michael Ciaramello and friends from the Pinellas Park Fire Department held a raffle for a Harley Davidson motorcycle, and on March 15, 1997, presented Robby with a check for $28,595. It appeared the Lord wanted us to continue our current course.

However, by April I was wondering if everything really would be alright. Another MRI on April 6 indicated an enlargement of the nodule that first appeared six weeks earlier. It had doubled in size. As the weeks went on, Robby's health began to decline. By the end of April he was sleeping most of the day. He also was back on Decadron, a steroid drug to control inflammation; it was the only way to control the severe headaches he was suffering. His eye began to cross again as well. That scared us. A crossed eye is how we found the beast to begin with. For whatever good the Antineoplastons did, they weren't enough to keep the monster away completely. It was growing uncharacteristically slow, but it was growing.

I had been at a new job for only a few months, forced to leave my last job because they had already grown tired of my need for flexibility in taking Robby to doctor visits. We needed the money but were afraid to leave Robby far from our care. So we managed to arrange for him to be watched by people we trusted. Between Rick, his mom, and my dad, someone who loved Robby was always with him while I was away.

I worked forty-five minutes from home. Fortunately Dad was only fifteen minutes from there. Every Friday I'd take Robby to Dad's and then go to work. One particular Friday, Dad was waiting for me at the door.

"I have something for you," he smiled.

I could see the paper in his hand. "What's that?"

"You're not opposed to having someone pray for Robby are you?"

Growing up, Dad wasn't a saintly example. Let's just say . . . he had issues. He and Mom divorced when I was twelve, and since then he had remarried and become "born again." My siblings and I jokingly referred to him as the holy roller of the family.

"No, Dad, I'm not opposed to someone praying for Robby. Why?"

I could sense his hesitance as he handed me the paper. I suppose he knew I was a little resistant to the kind of church he went to. It wasn't bad; it just wasn't for me. I had my doubts about miraculous healings taking place in prayer meetings.

I glanced at the title on the page: "Faith Outreach Center Presents 5 Miracle Services with Billy Burke."

"They're having a revival at our church next week. This preacher will be there praying for people. I was hoping you'd bring Robby."

I shrugged. "I don't know. I'll think about it."

Back in my van, I read the flyer in its entirety.

FAITH OUTREACH CENTER PRESENTS
5 MIRACLE SERVICES WITH

BILLY BURKE
SUNDAY APRIL 27 @ 6:00 PM
MONDAY-THURSDAY APRIL 28-MAY 1 @ 7:00 PM

HEALED AT AGE NINE OF TERMINAL BRAIN CANCER IN A KATHRYN KUHLMAN MEETING GOD HAS ANNOINTED HIM WITH THE HEALING GIFT.

HOSTS "THE MASTER'S TOUCH" TELEVISION PROGRAM ON CTN SATURDAY'S @ 8:00 PM

HE HAS HELD HEALING CRUSADES IN THE U.S.A., EUROPE, CARIBBEAN, AND CANADA.

TESTIMONIES OF MIRACULAOUS PHYSICAL HEALINGS, DEEP EMOTIONAL, AND MENTAL HEALINGS, AND DELIVERANCES FROM DEMONIC BONDAGES; ALL OCCUR REGULARLY IN BILLY'S MEETINGS.

"Healed at age nine of terminal brain cancer." Those words jumped off the page and repeated in my mind. I had been praying for an example, one person who had survived brain cancer. I just

needed one. If one person had made it, I knew we could too. Intrigued by the fact that this man claimed to have been healed of a brain tumor as a boy, I wondered, *Is this what you have in mind, Lord?*

Racing home from work the following Monday, I had little time to get dinner prepared before we had to leave. Dad's church was an hour away. As I hustled in the door, Rick's mom, Sharron, aka Nanu, greeted me.

"Hello, how was your day?"

"As good as it could be, I guess. How's Robby doing?"

"He's fine. Slept a lot today."

"Good, he'll be rested up for tonight."

The flyer Dad gave me hung on the refrigerator, and Sharron referred to it. "Ya' know, that's the guy I told you about."

"What guy? I don't know what you're talking about."

"Didn't Rick tell you?"

"No."

"Yeah, I saw this guy on television Saturday night. He prays for people and they get healed. I told Rick about it."

He must've forgotten about it, because I didn't have any idea what she was talking about. So she saw the guy on TV . . . big deal.

"Well, I don't know about that," I responded, "but Rick and I decided that it wouldn't hurt to have this pastor pray for Robby."

I actually thought it might do us good too. We hadn't been to church in months. With all the fund-raisers, work, and just trying to live, I hadn't much time for Bible reading either. But I still prayed, and I knew where my Bible was if I needed it.

Once Rick finally arrived, we rushed through dinner and waited anxiously for my mom to get there. Sharron was going with us. The church was supposed to provide nursery service, but I didn't want to leave my baby girl with strangers. I didn't know these people. She was only a year old. I had enough stress and didn't need something happening to her too.

When I'd called to ask Mom to babysit, she took me by surprise. "As long as you're considering going to that kind of thing"—I knew she didn't really approve—"a customer of mine told me about a place around here that does the same kind of thing."

"Oh really?" I asked. I wasn't interested in going to any other place like this. I had been to one other such meeting in a little church in a city close to ours. It was strange. The service was incredibly long and I'd felt really awkward. I never thought I'd be considering, much less going to, such a service again—but here we were.

"Yeah," Mom continued, "I guess they have healing services every month or something. He says that his pastor prays for people, and I guess a lot of them get healed."

"Well, let me get through this one, and I'll let you know if I'm interested."

Mom finally arrived to watch the kids. We said our hellos and good-byes as we ran out the door.

"The kids already ate," I explained as I rushed out. "Make sure they are in bed by eight."

As I hurried past, she handed me a piece of paper from a yellow sticky pad—scribbled writing filled both sides.

"Here are the directions to that place I told you about," Mom said.

I grabbed it and shoved it into my purse. "Yeah, yeah, okay . . . I'll look at it later. We're running late."

Somehow we arrived on time. We followed Dad and his wife, Rhonda, into the church. He chose the second row. I think he would've chosen the front row, but someone was already sitting there. I was a little uncomfortable and would've preferred to sit in the back. I was scared and didn't know what to expect. But Dad's confidence to sit in the front of the church impressed me. When I was a little girl, he forfeited attending church with the rest of the family, many times. When he was there, he was miserable. He preferred to sit in the back and did not participate. He didn't sing, didn't pray, and certainly didn't participate in communion. I think he went simply because Mom told him to. Now he was different.

This was a quaint church—not too big or too small. The pews faced a large stage-like platform. Elevated a few steps from the rest of the congregation, it was the focal point at the front of the sanctuary. At one end stood a large piano, drums, and guitars with room for the choir. At the other, three large chairs.

As the music began, I stood with the rest of the crowd. I had never heard these songs before. Not that it mattered. I hadn't sung in church in years. I don't know why, really. Maybe I was afraid someone would hear me. Maybe I didn't feel like it. Maybe it just didn't matter if I sang. All I know is that I didn't sing in church anymore.

People were clapping with the music, hooting and hollering, hands raised in the air. It was like some sort of strange celebration. Rick nudged me to sing, acknowledging the words on the screen in front of us. I shook my head no, deciding to clap to the music instead.

In time the atmosphere in the room began to change. I looked over to see my dad smiling and singing, joining in the celebration. My dad . . . singing!

If he can do it, then I surely can too, I thought.

I did my best to follow along with the words on the screen. The music was energizing, the most beautiful songs I had ever heard. I could feel the presence of God mysteriously fill the air.

Three men came out and stood near the three large chairs.

"There he is! There he is!" Sharron whispered excitedly in my ear as she slapped my left arm.

"There who is?"

"The guy on TV!"

Pastor Billy had blond hair and was dressed head to toe in white—white suit, white leather shoes, white everything.

Rick looked at me and rolled his eyes. Both of us wondered if we'd made a mistake.

We hadn't. Never had we been taught in church by someone as in touch with the current reality we were forced to live in. He gave real-world lessons that were useful and applicable. Most importantly, he instilled hope.

When he was finished teaching, Pastor Billy began to call people out for healing. A line began to form as more and more people stood for prayer. We watched for a while, not sure what to do, waiting to be convinced to go up. People were falling all over the place, referred to by the preacher as falling under the power of the

Holy Spirit. At times the floor was covered with people, some smiling, some crying, all evidently having some sort of spiritual encounter.

I remembered times, as a teenager, laughing at people getting slapped to the ground on TV. I had never seen it in person. But Pastor Billy didn't slap people to the ground; he gently touched them on the cheeks with both hands and they just fell. I was compelled to watch. At first, wondering if it was all real; ultimately, amazed at the things my eyes began to see.

It was well past 10:00 when the lady in front of us turned and told us to take Robby up in line. When only a couple of people remained, Rick stood up with Robby.

"Are you coming?" he asked.

I shook my head no. The look of fear on my face told him not to press it.

He rested Robby, now sleeping, on his shoulder and got in line.

"What's this? What's going on here?" the preacher asked Rick as they approached. I listened intently from my seat in the pew.

"My son has a brain tumor . . . cancer."

"How old is he?"

"Five."

"How long has he had this?"

"Uh . . . he already had one tumor removed last year. Now he's had a recurrence."

"What's the doctor say?"

"It's not good. They don't have much hope."

"Do you have a church?"

"Yes."

"Ya' do? Where do you go to church?"

"It's over in Pinellas County."

"Yeah? What's the name of it?"

"Uh, St. Patrick's. It's—"

"Yeah, I know all about it."

"Dear Jesus," the pastor began to pray. As he asked the Lord to heal this precious little boy, the entire congregation began to pray along with him. One woman began wailing and crying aloud, praying in Spanish. Others were praying in tongues. At least that's what I thought they were doing. I had heard talk about it, but never witnessed it.

I prayed too, *"Please Lord, let this be the night. Please heal my little boy and end this nightmare."*

The man in white reached out—one hand on Robby's head, the other on Rick's cheek. Rick stumbled backward. He reached out and touched them for a second time. Again Rick stumbled back. I was certain they would both be lying on the floor just like dozens of others I'd seen that night. Part of me wanted them to be. If they fell too, it must be real. But they didn't.

The preacher turned to walk away from them. Suddenly he spun around, faced toward them, and declared, "He'll be healed. Your son will be healed, but it won't be right away. It's going to be a process."

Processes take time, and that was something we were running out of. I wanted to believe in that moment, but why was it taking so long? The course of Robby's treatment had already taken nearly a year. I demanded to the heavens that he should be healed now. Why did others walk away that evening free from their bondages while we left still shackled with ours?

Realizing we needed to take a stand, I vowed to never give up. Our due season would eventually come. It was just a matter of time.

12
IS FAILURE AN OPTION?

As the red glow of the rockets flared amid jumbo clouds of smoke, the Odyssey *blasted out of Earth's atmosphere. Excitement filled the air as America witnessed its third mission to the moon. Inside the Apollo spacecraft, three brave astronauts risked all for the privilege of walking on the lunar surface, unaware of the changes in fortune about to transpire.*

Two days after launch, an explosion violently shook the capsule. The team within was safe and sound, but the vessel's exterior was severely damaged. The crew was now stranded, alone in the darkness of space. With limited electrical power and oxygen running low, the men helplessly awaited assistance from experts at home.

As the catastrophe unfolded, Mission Control rallied. The broken spacecraft newly assessed, Apollo 13's astronauts were considered doomed. The moon mission was abandoned for one of higher importance—the lives of the crew must be saved.

While the world's best scientists calculated, the lives of the astronauts hung in the balance, the odds of success against them. With the ship's heat shield critically damaged, how could they survive the inferno of reentry?

The entire country watched and waited, tensions rising—the final outcome had yet to be decided. Believing for the best, the flight

119

director announced, *"We've never lost an American in space. We're . . . not going to lose one on my watch!"*[1]

After the prayer service, I was electrified. I couldn't wait to ask Rick if he felt anything. As soon as we got in the van, I started. "So?"

"So what?" Rick asked.

"What did it feel like?"

"I don't know how to describe it. I never felt anything like that before."

"What does that mean?"

"You'll just have to find out for yourself."

My eyes widened with fear and I shook my head rapidly, "Uh-uh."

"Yeah, I think you should," he teased.

"Come on. Seriously, I want to know if you felt anything."

"Well, when he put his hand on the right side of my face, it just lit up like a fire. It didn't hurt," he shrugged, "it felt good."

"Really?"

Rick nodded.

"I thought for sure you were going to fall."

"No way, man. I made up my mind before I got up there that I was *not* going to fall."

"You looked like you were going to fall."

"What are you talking about?"

"You stumbled backward when he touched you. I thought you were going to fall."

"No, I didn't."

"Yes, you did," his mother interjected.

The hour ride home gave us plenty of time to talk about the evening's events. All of us were excited and intrigued.

Rick's mom, Sharron, really enjoyed Billy Burke's preaching. "I'd love to go to his church someday," she said.

"Me too," I replied.

"I wonder where it is."

"Well, it has to be in Florida."

"How do you know that?"

"Because he was talking about the weather and he said when you live in Florida, like we do, ya' get spoiled."

"Oh yeah, that's right. But that could be anywhere. I wonder how we could find out what city it's in," Sharron said.

"Look in the book we bought. Maybe it says something in there," I advised her.

The dimness of the dome light did little to help her farsighted vision as she scanned the back cover of the book looking for an address.

"There's just a post office box address. It's in Clearwater," she replied.

"Maybe his church is in Clearwater. Does it say the name of the church anywhere?"

"Oh, here it is . . . Miracle Center World Outreach in Largo, Florida."

"Largo? It's right in our hometown?"

"That's what it says."

"I've never heard of it."

"Me neither," Rick said. "Let's look it up when we get home. Maybe we can go there Sunday."

Once we were home and the kids were in bed, we began our search for the church address. First we tried the yellow pages. We looked under every Christian denomination, but couldn't find it. Then we tried the white pages. No church listed as Miracle Center there either. Frustrated we were about to give up, when . . .

"Hold on a minute, I have an idea," I said. From my purse I retrieved the note Mom had given me earlier in the evening. I returned to the dining room table, reading the scribbled letters on the tiny piece of paper.

Looking up at Rick, I smiled, "Honey, I think God wants us to go this church."

"Let me see that," he said, grabbing the paper from my hands.

"What is it?" his mother asked.

"There it was the whole time . . . right in my purse."

"There what was?" she asked again.

Rick laid the note on the table in front of us. On it were step-by-step directions to the Miracle Center church. I thought about the name for a moment. The Miracle Center seemed the perfect place to go. We needed a miracle.

The next morning Robby woke up and walked out to the living room to greet me, "Mommy, I'm hungry."

I looked down to see my little boy's sleepy eyes staring up at me. "Oh my God, come here."

Robby came closer, his eyes questioning mine.

I caressed his cheeks in my hands, staring into his soft blue eyes. Smiling, I kissed his face over and over. "How do you feel?"

"Fine," he giggled.

I picked him up and squeezed him tight. "I think it's time for some tickle medicine."

He squealed with delight as I wrestled him to the ground and tickled him for several minutes.

After getting his breakfast and taking care of the other two children, I called Rick. "Did you look at Robby's eye this morning before you left?"

"No, he was half asleep. I changed his IV bags, asked him if he was okay, and turned on the cartoon channel for him. Why? Is something wrong?"

"No."

"What is it then?"

"Well, I was going to wait until you got home . . . but I can't wait."

"What is it?"

"His eyes are straight."

"No way. Really? You're not playing a trick on me, are you?"

"No, really, his eyes are perfectly straight and he's awake. He's been awake for three hours now."

"I can't believe that," he replied enthusiastically.

"Do you think last night had anything to do with it?"

"I don't know."

"Maybe the cancer is gone."

"I don't know, Les. Remember? The pastor said it was going to be a process."

"Oh yeah," I responded, disappointed.

"Yeah, when he said that, I thought, *What kind of crap is that?*"

"Well, I hope the process is a quick one."

"Me too. Give Robby a kiss for me. I'll try to get home early."

Later that day, Rick ran in the house, full of excitement. "Robby's outside playing," he called out.

"Yes, I know," I answered.

"When I was driving up the street I saw this little boy running and playing, and I was thinking how great that would be if it were Robby. Then I pulled up to the driveway and it was him!"

"I know. Isn't it wonderful?"

I hoped this meant Robby was healed, yet I still couldn't help but wonder how much longer he'd be with us. I wanted this journey to be over, but my gut told me there was more to endure.

Something changed in me after that meeting at my father's church. Adorned in a dress and heels, my scrubs intentionally forgotten at home, I arrived at work already prepared for the exciting evening ahead.

Chad, one of the guys I worked with, noticed my new dress code. "What are you all dressed up for?"

"I'm going to church."

"Yeah," he laughed, "sure you are."

"Are you saying someone like me would never go to church?"

He laughed hysterically. "Really, why are you all dressed up?"

"I told you, I'm going to church tonight after work." I smiled, knowing I would never convince him.

Ever since that first healing service, I was addicted. Being in the presence of God felt indescribably good and I wanted to be near Him as much as I could. Given that I had yet to learn how to create that experience myself, I began going to Miracle Center services regularly. I knew I could find Him there.

Robby's eye didn't cross anymore, but the beast in his brain continued to grow, and in June 1997, Robby underwent his second craniotomy. I hated that he had to have his skull cracked open again, but the tumor had grown exponentially, now 3.2 centimeters. Better to get it out before it spread.

At least I wasn't scared this time. I believed that Jesus would heal Robby someday. I kept reminding myself that it was a process. I didn't understand His reasons for putting us through this again, but I tried my best to trust Him.

Having experienced one eight-hour brain surgery, we settled into the waiting room with several new friends from Miracle Center. Instead of fret and worry, we shared stories of things the Lord had done in our lives, spurring quite a bit of laughter.

One of the associate pastors from my mother's church was there also. We met Laura in the early days of this journey, right after Robby's initial surgery. I remember when she first came to meet us. She was young, quiet and soft-spoken, struggling for the right thing to say. I knew she didn't believe me then when I told her Robby was going to be fine. Now here she was, laughing and sharing stories too.

As we sat and talked, I felt compelled to share my experience at the cathedral a year earlier. Unsure how I'd be received, I told my small group of new friends of my encounter with Jesus.

"I believe you," Laura piped up.

I was surprised to hear her speak first. She was so timid when I first met her. A pastor at a modest Methodist church, Laura was the last one in the group that I expected to be so enthusiastic.

She continued, "I've had a similar experience myself."

Sharing her story, Laura took on a brightness and confidence that I hadn't seen in her before. As we listened, the group oozed gratitude and excitement. With others sharing their own divine experiences, I knew I was not alone.

"Laura, I am so happy to hear that you are such a strong believer in divine intervention," I said when she finished. "I would've never guessed that, especially the first time we met you. We didn't know you were an associate pastor. You were so quiet and shy. We thought you were just some rookie prayer-team member."

The group laughed.

"You know," Laura replied, "I wouldn't have told you my experience, but you shared that story and you seem so convinced that God is going to heal Robby—"

"What are you trying to say?"

"The reason I was so quiet when I met you the first time is because when they found out I was there to visit you . . . and . . . I guess they saw my clergy badge . . . they raced up to me and said, 'Thank God you're here!' . . . I was taken by surprise." She shifted in her seat, leaning forward, whispering, "They told me that you thought he was going to be fine, but they said, 'He's not leaving this hospital alive.' They told me I needed to talk some sense into you. And then, well, I got in the room and you were so convinced that he was going to get better . . ."

"I see."

". . . I didn't know what to say."

"They never told us that, not in so many words, anyhow. Well, I'm glad we all know now that they were wrong." I winked.

We weren't the least surprised when a nurse came out about an hour and a half later. We knew the drill—hourly reports until surgery was finished.

After locating us the nurse informed, "The surgery is over."

Rick and I both jumped to our feet.

"What?" I asked.

"What's wrong?" Rick echoed.

The smiles on the faces of family and friends quickly fell into grief and concern.

"Nothing's wrong," the nurse assured. "Robby is doing well. The tumor is out and Dr. Solomon is finishing closing him up."

The group of us gave a collective sigh of relief.

"But you've only been in there a little over an hour," I said. "Last time . . ."

"Dr. Solomon will be out in a little while to go over everything with you," she answered.

When he joined us, Dr. Solomon described the tumor as uncharacteristic for medulloblastoma. Normally mushy and gelatinous, this tumor was hard and fibrous. To us, this meant the Antineoplastons had some sort of effect (though Dr. Solomon didn't mention it), but biopsy confirmed that it was indeed a recurrence of medulloblastoma.

Unlike Robby's first hospitalization, the surgery was brief, recovery quick, and no complications. He was discharged exactly two weeks from his admission date.

For weeks after, Rick and I agonized over what to do next. Local doctors continued to advise radiation and chemo. We didn't want to do anything. Postoperative testing showed no sign of cancer anywhere.

Eventually, fear of yet another recurrence convinced us to get a compassionate exception from the FDA to use Antineoplastons for preventative use.

Sadly, an MRI only a few months later, in October 1997, showed abnormal growth in Robby's brain. This time there were three tumors.

What could we do now? The fund was practically empty, not that it mattered. The FDA wouldn't permit us to use Antineoplastons again, even if we wanted to. We were convinced that a higher dose would be effective, but Robby's small body couldn't handle the fluid volume necessary to deliver a high enough dose of the life-saving medication. For all the others it worked for, it ultimately wasn't enough to cure Robby. We were grateful for Dr. Burzynski and his treatment. It bought Robby time to become a normal boy again. I had no regrets, certain that any other path would've led quickly to his demise.

Now we had to find a different way. Learning of a Catholic priest who was said to have the gift of healing, we took Robby once again for prayer. It made sense. After all, it was a Catholic cathedral in which I personally encountered Jesus.

After mass, people lined up to receive prayer. Rick and I took Robby up together.

The priest gently asked, "What is wrong here?"

Rick answered, "Brain cancer."

He tenderly laid his hands upon Robby's head and began to pray. Suddenly a sound of electricity—like mosquitoes hitting a bug zapper—emerged from the priest.

"ZZZZZ . . . ZZZZZ . . . ZZZZZ."

Three times the zapping electrical sound buzzed. I wondered how he knew. We hadn't told him there were three tumors.

The priest opened his eyes and looked at Rick. "He will be healed," he stated reassuringly. "He will be healed."

He smiled at Robby. "Jesus has big plans for you."

Now we'd heard it twice—two ministers, two different denominations, but the same Jesus. I wanted to believe him. But what if?

What if they're still there? What if the tumors keep growing back? What if I'm crazy? What if I've gotten my hopes up for nothing? What if I'm wrong? What if he dies?

I was what-ifing myself right back to a place of doubt and fear. I hadn't been scared like this since the first minutes I'd heard Robby had a brain tumor.

In the midst of my "what if" ceremony, God's voice emerged. *"What if? What if you aren't crazy? What if things go well? What if Robby does get healed? Why aren't you asking these things?"*

I swiftly realized there was another side to the "what if" game. "Good question," I replied.

"Whatsoever things are true, whatsoever things are honest, whatsoever things are just, whatsoever things are pure, whatsoever things are lovely, whatsoever things are of good report . . . think on these things."[2]

Robby had his third resection on October 13, 1997. Before surgery, we presented Dr. Solomon with a Christian CD to play during the operation. He jokingly let us know that it would be best if we let him listen to his country music during the surgery, no need for distraction. But he agreed to play our CD in the operating room during the prep time.

"Dr. Solomon," Rick asked, "we were about to pray before Robby goes into surgery. Would you pray with us?"

He politely declined. "But I want you to know that I pray before every surgery. It's a little Jewish prayer . . ."

Rick and I smiled at each other.

". . . called the Shema, and it goes like this: 'Hear O Israel, the Lord is our God; the Lord is one.' It's an old, old prayer that comes from the Old Testament. Then, on top of that, I add a prayer asking the Lord to protect the child."

Rick smiled. "That's good," he nodded, "it'll do." He winked at me.

Smiling, I nodded in agreement.

Regrettably, the tumors hadn't magically disappeared and they needed to be removed. Surgery went well and Robby was discharged a short week later. Even though his recurrences seemed to get worse each time, his recoveries were quicker. God was still in this, but how much more did He expect us to endure?

Running out of treatment options, we decided to give Duke another chance. We were hesitant to do anything drastic, and thus Robby started with three rounds of oral chemotherapy. This drug, called VP-16, can sometimes hold off new growth. Following this would be the stem-cell rescue we had discussed on our first visit. I didn't know if that's what God wanted us to do or not. The heavens were quiet. At least it would buy us more time while we waited for further direction.

Unfortunately, the next MRI, less than three months later in January 1998, indicated recurrence with metastatic disease present in the brain. Now there were several areas affected. The VP-16 wasn't touching it. The beast was getting stronger, and coming back quicker.

Again I researched the Internet, hoping to find something new. Indeed I did. A U.S. citizen, now living in the Dominican Republic, cured himself of a glioma (aggressive brain cancer) using a magnetic therapy he developed. He owned clinics in Europe, Mexico, and the Dominican Republic. The supporting rationale and science made sense, so I was willing to give it a try. I knew that surviving stem-cell rescue would be risky for Robby. I'd do anything to avoid it.

I discussed the possibility with Dr. Longee. He seemed to understand my frustration and desperation, but he couldn't advocate our trying this alternative treatment. Though when pressed about the risks of waiting a few more weeks before pursuing the stem-cell rescue, he answered, "If you're going to try anything else, do it now before it's too late."

Rick took out a loan against his pension. We made travel arrangements and were quickly on our way out of the country for one last desperate attempt to cure our son.

The Apollo 13 mission was dubbed a "successful failure." Though the astronauts returned safely to Earth, they never made it to the moon. We too seemed to fail at every attempt in our mission to find a cure for our son. Would this fail also? Could success somehow be found in the midst of our failures? I wasn't certain, but I pressed on, knowing, in the immortal words of Apollo Flight Director Gene Kranz, "Failure is not an option."[3]

13
LIGHT

It was a simpler time, when horse and buggy were all a family needed for occasional travels, when newly connected telegraph lines were considered high tech, and when the fall of night overtaking day was the norm. People then didn't realize how constrained they were by traveling difficulties, slow communication methods, and limited hours of daylight.

They had no radios, no television, and no automobiles. No one had ever heard of airplanes, motion pictures, phonographs, or even light bulbs. The world was confined by darkness, silence, and immobility.

But it would not stay that way for long—for on February 11, 1847, in a little brick house in the hills of Milan, Ohio, Thomas Alva Edison was born. Young Thomas took a strong interest in the sciences and grew to dream of the day when light would overtake the darkness of night.

Light is the fastest thing in the universe, yet cannot be touched or felt. A mere eight minutes is all it needs to travel to Earth from the sun. Edison toiled laboriously to harness it, with visions of bringing his invention into every home.

We cannot see without it—merely the translation of an electrical signal from the brain converted from its beams, light is all our eyes really see. Guiding us from the darkest of places, it emerges as a saving hand. Though we may stumble in the darkness, in the light we always find our way.[1]

The two-hour flight took us over the waters of the Atlantic Ocean to the small island nation of the Dominican Republic. Staring down from the window of the plane, I could see the tiny airport below. The small airfield with its one measly runway was isolated on the southernmost end of the island. *That's it?* I wondered to myself with mild disbelief. As I eyed the gorgeous blue water crashing on the edges of the land below, my mind briefly explored the extremes to which we were willing to go. *I sure hope we're doing the right thing.*

Except for a trip to Niagara Falls I took as a child, we'd never been outside of the United States. Third-world countries were something we'd seen only on TV.

Entering the Santo Domingo airport, we quickly realized this place was more foreign than we could have ever dreamed. Even though it was January, the hot, humid air of the tropics nearly took my breath away as I entered the jet bridge to the gate. The terminal was dingy and the lighting noticeably dim. On the plane, everyone spoke English, but now we were in the minority.

Certain that my dear husband would be very uncomfortable with the language barrier (remember, he wanted everyone in America to speak English), my mind instantly pondered ways to help him cope. A local firm called Family & Friends was providing our ground transportation. We expected to see them when we got off of the plane, but none of the chauffer signs bore our name. *Uh-oh. I can see this is going to be more difficult than I thought.*

I began wondering what kind of horrible mistake we'd made, but didn't want to let on to the rest of my family. *Be strong,* I encouraged myself. Unsure where to go next, we followed the flow of the mob funneling through the gates.

Again I questioned if we'd made the right decision. I mean, we prayed, doors opened, we walked through. The situation was desperate and the timing critical. I couldn't wait for divine confirmation, so . . . here we were. Concern was plastered across

Rick's face. I knew there was no quick fix for our new dilemma—best to proceed as planned.

How bad can it get? I thought.

Trying to make light of the situation, I turned to Rick and smiled. "We're not in Kansas anymore, Toto," I said, laughing.

"You're telling me," he grumbled.

Crowded in on all sides, people pushed us forward, approaching some sort of immigration window. The lady inside yelled at me in Spanish.

"Habla Inglés?" I asked.

"Qué?

"English?"

"No. Gaba digaba gaba," she jabbered on.

It was all gibberish to me. I tried handing her the papers given to us on the plane—something we were to keep with us at all times. She shook her head indignantly, stamped the back of our papers, and waved us through—yelling even more.

We continued to follow the crowd toward the baggage claim area, found our bags, and headed toward customs. Bright yellow lines painted on the floor boldly delineated the difference between international and Dominican land. We hesitated before them momentarily—allowing the possibility of turning around to linger in our minds for one more second—then crossed over.

Everyone in the large room was speaking only Spanish and they were doing it *very* loudly. There were five lanes with an agent manning every one. All of them yelled in Spanish as passengers flung their suitcases onto the rollers to be inspected. Aggressively the agents tore through each piece of luggage—flinging, emptying, leaving nothing unturned.

We cautiously approached the area. Then something caught our eye, stopping us dead in our tracks.

"Oh crap," Rick whispered.

On the wall behind the inspection area, twenty-plus men in military dress stood at attention, machine guns by their sides.

He was obviously thinking the same thing I was. Our luggage contained medicine and needles. We'd hurriedly fled the U.S., trying to give our son a shot at a potential cure, our other children brought with us to keep our family together. Now, visions of a Spanish-yelling customs agent carting us off to jail—with our children going to God knows where—began to flash through my mind as we stared at the chaos.

With Amanda in my arms, the five of us stood shoulder to shoulder, paralyzed by fear.

I glanced down at Ricky and Robby, huddled close to us with uncertainty in their eyes. I didn't want to scare them, but I was scared myself and looked to my husband, expecting him to know what to do.

Terrified, I whispered, "What do we do?"

Rick shrugged. "I don't know," he whispered back.

A man in a customs uniform waved us toward a line. We stood still, staring forward, unable to move.

Then a female customs agent waved us to her line, calling out in Spanish. I couldn't understand a word. Slowly we edged toward her. An uneasy feeling had me speculating what would happen next. Rick lifted up a suitcase to set it upon the roller-lined shelf for her to examine.

"No! No! No!" she yelled.

My heart beat faster and faster. *We are going to mess this up and end up in a third-world prison,* I thought.

The female customs agent began gibbering more and waving for us to go through. Again we stood helpless, staring at the men with guns lined against the wall, afraid to make a move.

"Is okay, is okay," she said in broken English.

We looked toward the soldiers. My heart raced while our feet stood firmly still, unable to move for fear of what would happen next. We turned back to look at the female customs agent. Every person who had approached those lanes had been thoroughly inspected. No one else was waved through.

"Is okay," she said, smiling.

We inched our way past her, half expecting to be stopped again. Once through we breathed a sigh of relief for another door opened—literally.

Bit by bit we moved toward the door, noticing that no one was allowed to return inside once they exited. We had no idea what was on the other side. Peeking out, we saw hundreds of Dominicans crowded outside.

Rick, clearly annoyed by our new prospects, looked at me. "What the heck?"

I shrugged my shoulders and shook my head. I was wondering the same thing myself.

As we peered outside, the large crowd of people yelled frantically in Spanish, climbing over one another trying to get our attention. We had no idea what they were saying—they certainly were a scary sight. After trading a U.S. dollar for Dominican coins, I called Family & Friends from a pay phone inside the airport.

"They say our driver is waiting outside," I told Rick.

"You stay here with the kids. I'll go look," he instructed.

I stood close to the exit doors, trying not to make eye contact with the soldiers who stood only a few feet away.

My heart beat frantically. *I wish he'd hurry*, I thought.

A few minutes later, Rick appeared outside the exit. "Come on, I found our ride."

"Thank God!"

Loading into the minivan outside, we were welcomed by two friendly guides who spoke English. We drove down the long road toward the city with my senses taking in all of the new sights, sounds, and smells. The air was thick with the heavy scent of diesel. The street was lined with trash, large chunks of cement covered in graffiti, and beat up cars evidently dumped by the side of the road. *Oh my, what have we done?* I asked myself. The images flashing past were reminiscent of scenes I had witnessed only on TV from coverage of the Gulf War. I tried hard to suppress the fear and guilt I was feeling, believing that this treatment offered hope, and knowing we could always go home if things weren't what we expected.

It was dark by the time we checked into our hotel. Everything is scarier in the dark.

It was difficult adapting to our new living arrangements. Our first hotel was small, smelly, and eerie. For four days, the kids and I stayed locked in our room; Rick would venture out to find a place to trade currency and get food—which was expensive. We weren't sure we'd have enough money to survive the four to six weeks that Robby needed treatment.

Though miserable, I took comfort every night in the view. Out our window we could see the lighted cross in the sky—beamed up from the Columbus lighthouse. The people of this nation were devout Christians who outwardly demonstrated their love of Christ at every opportunity. In the weeks to come we became quite adept at living in a third-world country, having learned enough Spanish to get by.

Gathered daily in the clinic waiting area, we met people from all over the world, each seeking hope from an unproven treatment. There were men and women of all ages and ethnicities, farmers, senators, children—even the pastor from a Hutterite community (a branch off the Amish) in Canada.

For four weeks we washed our clothes every day in the tub, boiled our drinking water, and made do trying to eat healthy in a land of poverty and lack. At home we were barely middle class, but in Santo Domingo we were rich Americans! Our small, 1,200-square-foot house in Florida was a mansion for the people here, most of whom lived in homes no larger than our toolshed. No furniture crowded the dirt floors of their homes, and there were no doors or windows to keep out insects and rodents, yet these people took pride in their living spaces. Humbled, we became grateful for the privileges we were born into.

In Santo Domingo, crime was low. Men armed with machine guns secured business and home alike. Here it was okay to shoot those who committed a crime against you. In spite of this, we learned to feel safe. They *loved* Americans.

Morning through afternoon, every weekday was spent at the clinic. Many of the other patients were doing well. But Robby got worse. His first MRI indicated an enlargement of the mass.

The doctor said, "Not to worry. 'Tis sign of tumor breakdown. Is no problem."

It didn't sound right, but we continued to pray and trust.

After Robby's treatment each day, we returned to our hotel in late afternoon. Reserving our money for necessities, there was little to do to pass the remaining hours of the day. The hotel had a pool, which we enjoyed when it wasn't full of ash from the generator outside. We purchased books and puzzles to keep the children entertained, and found one or two cable channels beamed from the U.S. At night Rick frequently spent time riding the elevator with Emmanuel.

Emmanuel was the hotel elevator operator. The typical electric elevator did not require an advanced technician to push its buttons, but he was there to serve. A native of Santo Domingo, Emmanuel spoke seven languages and happily taught the children Español during our rides with him. Nearly every night, Bible in hand, Rick would ride the elevator and talk with Emmanuel for hours.

On weekends we ventured around the city to avoid the temptation of lying around our tiny one-room living quarters. Plus, going to some of the tourist sights made us feel like a normal family. Amazingly, there was quite a bit to see. Our first weekend there, eight of us jammed into a five-passenger Toyota Corolla for the two-hour trip into the mountains—one place where the splendor of God is greatly evident.

Subsequent weekends we were invited to dine with the director of Youth With A Mission and taken to the national zoo and aquarium by new friends. I even tried an all-day shopping trip with the gals to Mercado Modelo.

We were in the oldest city in the Western world—rich in history. By our fifth weekend, we were comfortable getting around the city and decided to have a homeschool field trip to both the castle and the palace of Christopher Columbus. We found a relatively inexpensive tour guide who took us to the first churches built in the western hemisphere—the first Catholic cathedral and the first Protestant church. Then we toured the castle of Christopher Columbus . . . interesting but *creepy*.

Robby's energy level had declined significantly in recent days, so Rick carried him through all our destinations that day. He intermittently slept on his father's shoulder, and by noon it became obvious that Robby was not up to the outing. We returned to our room for a nap.

Later Robby awoke from his sleep, crying.

"Robby, what's the matter, pumpkin?" Rick asked.

Robby began holding his head and screaming in pain.

"Do you have a headache?" I asked. My heart sunk in my chest as I suppressed the panic inside.

One of the doctors made a house call to the hotel. "There is no way to tell what is the problem without MRI," he told us.

"I think we're going to go home," Rick said.

"I think is okay. We can get MRI on Monday."

"That's two days away," Rick argued.

"Yes, you must make decision. But I think is okay to wait for MRI," he encouraged.

Why was this happening again? Why didn't anything we tried work? We did our best to follow God's plan for us. Why was He letting this happen?

It was already Saturday evening, and impossible to get a flight out at this point. We called the airline to see if anything was available for Sunday. There were no open seats available on Sunday and only two seats on Monday. If we were to take Robby home, only one of us could go. The other would have to wait in Santo Domingo with Ricky and Amanda until the next available flight.

"Which of us will go with him?" I asked Rick. I was afraid to travel with Robby alone. *How would I make the six-hour drive home from the Miami airport with Robby getting sick the entire time?* Going home alone scared me—partly because I'd worry about the rest of my family being stuck in another country far from home. But mostly because I didn't want to deal with the doctors and the hospital and the decisions and . . . the truth is—I really thought I might have to face Robby's demise alone. I couldn't bear the thought of it.

"I'm not leaving you here alone with the kids," Rick insisted.

"Let's just wait 'til Monday. We can't get a flight out before then anyway," I begged.

"I guess we have no choice."

Our family prayed together that night. "Heavenly Father," Rick led, "we need You now more than ever. Please show us the way. If You want us to stay, please give us assurance and peace. If it's time to go home, please make a way."

We spent the evening cuddling with the kids, every moment together newly appreciated and cherished.

Hours later I awoke to the sound of Robby vomiting. Rick, sleeping in bed next to him, was rapidly up at his side. We medicated Robby for his headache and cleaned the mess. I knew what this meant—both of us did. Rick's eyes stared desperately into mine as we gleaned each other's thoughts.

"It's only 4 a.m.," I said. "The airlines aren't open yet."

"Start packing, we're getting out of here today."

"But there aren't any seats available today."

"I don't care. We'll sit at the airport until we can get a flight."

The two of us raced around the room shoving everything into suitcases. At exactly 7:00 a.m., I called the airline.

Rick, just out of the shower, asked, "Well?"

"We can all get on a flight, but it leaves at nine."

"The airport is forty-five minutes away."

Unable to hide my worry, I shook my head, "I don't know if we can get a ride to the airport with this short notice."

"Do it," Rick commanded.

I immediately called Family & Friends, who, in spite of it being time to transport patients to clinic, had a van available.

Crowded in the minivan once again, I stared out the window as the deep-blue water whizzed by. The white caps of the waves crashed beautifully upon the jagged rocks of the shore. Though I was looking forward to being home again, a piece of me regretted leaving this place, especially this way.

I gazed up to the sky, praying all would be well, and saw two birds glide into view, reviving happy memories of times past. I smiled, remembering whenever a white dove appeared to me during tough times, it encouraged me to press on. But this time my hopes fell as I focused up in the sky and realized the black bird was *chasing* the white one. Grieving, I watched as the dark one gained ground, tormenting the white bird in flight. I didn't want the dark side to win.

We slipped effortlessly through customs and made it onto the plane, an absolute miracle. Less than twenty-four hours earlier, there were no seats available for that day. Now we had five *and* they were all together. Not just five but six! An entire row at the back of the plane was seemingly set aside for us, with room for Robby to lie down using two seats.

Eventually the water beneath us disappeared and Miami came into view. *We're home. Thank You, God!* An unexpected flood of relief washed over me and I understood for the first time why people get off planes and kiss the ground upon returning home from a foreign place. I had the urge to do the same.

It was nearly ten o'clock when we pulled into our driveway. Why were we always arriving at our destinations in the dark? Though Robby's condition continued to decline, we decided to keep him home and deal with the hospital in the morning. *They aren't going to do anything tonight anyway,* I reasoned. Robby slept peacefully between Rick and me. Snuggled up to my little boy, sleep evaded as I tearfully prayed, afraid this would be the last night he ever slept at home.

At the hospital the next morning, the doctors were curt with us. They ran some tests and told us there was a recurrence with some spread in the brain. We were disappointed, but not surprised—we'd been through this enough times to recognize the symptoms. Now we waited for them to decide what they were going to do next. After several hours, the ER doctor came with a decision.

"We're going to admit him," he informed us in an annoyed tone.

"Okay," I responded.

"Dr. Solomon will operate tomorrow to place a shunt."

"A shunt? Why is he doing that?" I asked. I was really surprised. I thought for sure they would be scheduling surgery to remove the tumors. Questions raced through my mind. *Are they going to place a shunt for comfort measures only? Will they even try to save him?*

"Because your son's head is full of tumor, and his intracranial pressure is through the roof!" he shouted at me.

Somehow I remained calm. I looked at Rick with a "Can you believe this?" kind of look, stunned at the doctor's aggressiveness. He'd never met us before that day. Though unhappy with the way he treated us, a part of me felt I deserved it. I was weary from years of fighting, but I couldn't let go yet. Certain the doctors were going to take their frustration with us and our lack of following their orders out on Robby, I feared they were giving up on him again and it was all my fault. I just needed them to forgive me so they would still try to save Robby.

I turned back toward the doctor. "I realize that," I calmly replied, "but he's never done that before. Why isn't he doing the resection?"

"He's booked. Can't do it until next week."

"But it can grow exponentially by then."

"Well, you should've thought about that before and followed your doctor's advice." His words jabbed at my heart.

I hung my head in shame. *Maybe he's right,* I thought. *If we'd done everything correctly, we wouldn't be here now.* This latest MRI indicated several affected areas in his brain, with spread to the spine. I didn't understand why Dr. Solomon was waiting so long. Robby's condition was declining rapidly. One more week could be fatal.

The next day we waited with Robby as he lay sleeping in ICU. Dr. Solomon's partner, Dr. T, stopped in to check on us. In the past he had made it clear how he felt about our involvement in Robby's treatment plans. My mind traveled back in time to one such conversation.

"You ask too many questions!" Dr. T roared. "You should just stop asking questions. Stop trying to figure everything out for yourself and leave it up to someone who knows what they're doing!"

I'd sat back in my chair. Smiling, I stared firmly into his eyes. Slowly I turned my gaze up toward heaven and held it there a few moments. With the smile still firmly affixed to my face, my gaze returned toward the doctor. I nodded. "I am," I replied.

But that was a year ago, and today the angry feelings shared in that argument didn't matter anymore. For whatever disagreements we'd had before, Robby's current state pushed it all aside. Now the look on Dr. T's face indicated his concern. "I can do the surgery," he said. "I can do it right now."

Silent, I looked to my husband.

Over the past two years, we had grown to love and respect Dr. Solomon. Not only could we trust his work ethic, but there were rare moments when his softer side prevailed and tiny cracks in his armor allowed us glimpses of his humanity. He really cared.

Rick shook his head. "That's alright," he replied. "We'll wait for Dr. Solomon."

Robby's vital signs were now the lowest they'd ever been. He no longer awoke for us, responding only to painful stimuli. His ribs poked out of his tiny chest, which rattled noisily as he inhaled short quick breaths; long periods of stillness stretched in between. His pulse and blood pressure continued downward.

Working many years with the elderly, I recognized this condition. The doctors and nurses, once reactively racing to improve his condition, now walked slowly. They recognized it too. The long fight was over. Robby had lived six years, three months, and twelve days in our charge. Staring silently at his little hands, I grasped tightly onto one, leaned over and gently kissed his little face. My eyes wandered across his small body; his skin wrapped tightly over his protruding little bones. The once playful, energetic body that housed his spirit now resembled a refugee camp victim.

Darkness was closing in on us all, and I couldn't do a thing to stop it. I just sat there, unable to move or even think. Numb, I had no more tears, no more courage, and no more fear. I was defeated—there was nothing more I could do.

I give up, Lord. I prayed silently. *I give up.* We'd reached a threshold. Our world was about to radically change, whether we liked it or not; might as well surrender. *I've done everything I can. I just can't do any more.* More love could never flow from a mother's heart. There was only one thing left to say—*he's in Your hands now. It's all up to You.*

During Robby's first surgery, I thought I handed him over to God. This time . . . I knew I did. His needs were far beyond my abilities.

I couldn't imagine what life would be like without Robby. I may have been willing to die for him, but I didn't need to—someone else already had. Robby was His son too, and no matter how much I loved Robby, I could never love him like Jesus. His love burns brighter than all the stars in the heavens combined, and in His light, darkness cannot survive.

14
POWER OF WATER

"Ha ha ha ha," the wicked witch cackled, "Well! Ring around the rosy—a pocket full of spears!" The evil sorceress approached her four captives. "Thought you'd be pretty foxy, didn't you? Well! The last to go will see the first three go before her!" She cackled devilishly, "and your mangy little dog too!"

The wicked witch walked over to a fiery torch mounted on the wall. Lifting the end of her broom, she ignited the bristles. "How about a little fire, Scarecrow?" she asked. Reaching out with her flaming stick, she touched it upon Scarecrow's arm.

"No! No! Help!! I'm burning!" Scarecrow yelled.

Dorothy screamed.

"I'm burning! I'm burning! Help! Help!" Scarecrow pled.

With the best of intentions, Dorothy reached for a nearby bucket of water.

The witch yelled, "Don't throw that water!"

But it was too late—caught in the cross fire, she was doused as well.

"Ahhhhhh!" she screamed. "You cursed brat! Look what you've done! I'm melting! Melting!" The witch's stature rapidly declined as she shouted, "Oh, what a world! What a world! Who would have thought a good little girl like you could destroy my beautiful wickedness!?" She screamed and wailed violently until nothing was left of her, "I'm going . . . ohhhhhh! Oh!"[1]

143

Water is a prevalent force throughout all aspects of life. It cools in the heat of a summer's day, provides purification from pollutants, and quenches our thirst. This simple chemical substance is essential to all life, yet has a life of its own.

This same refreshing liquid that provides a multitude of benefits also has the power to carve rock, sink ships, and destroy cities . . . washing away everything caught in its intense path—even evil.

Having the shunt placement allowed for better movement of Robby's cerebrospinal fluid and was supposed to make him "pop right back." But it didn't . . . not really. At home, waiting for yet another surgery, at least he would wake up now, and his headaches were much improved, but he still had no energy. Rather than play, he lay around and slept most of the time.

A week after the shunt placement, Robby had his fourth craniotomy. Before discharge, Dr. Cotman came to visit again. Radiation was still the recommended course of treatment. I sat and listened as Rick and Dr. Cotman discussed the procedures and potential side effects. It was nauseating listening to all of the bad things that could happen.

In the middle of their "grim fest," I stood to my feet. "Dr. Cotman, are these side effects definite or just possible?"

"Well, I have to go over all of them with you because they are all possible. And in most cases, many of these will be present."

I stared in thought for a moment, then looked back at him and replied, "I just need to know one thing. Is it possible to go through radiation without any of these symptoms?"

He chuckled, "It's highly unlikely, but . . . anything is possible."

"That's all I needed to know."

Robby recovered quickly from this surgery. So well, in fact, he was discharged home after only three days. At Dr. Solomon's office, a week later, Robby had his staples removed and we prepared for the final post-op MRI report.

"Hello, folks," Dr. Solomon greeted us.

"Hello," Rick and I responded in unison.

"Hi, Robby, how are you doing?"

"Fine," Robby answered.

"How has he been doing?"

"He's been fine," I stated.

"I . . . uh . . . I have the post-op scans here." Dr. Solomon turned to place them on the screen like he'd done many times before. "There's something on here that I wasn't expecting."

Rick and I looked at him questioningly.

"Well . . . let me just show it to you."

My heart skipped a beat. Robby already had multiple tumors in his head and spread to the spine before surgery. What more could there be?

The doctor flipped on the light switch and began pointing out the areas where he had removed tumors. "You see these two spots right here?" he asked, pointing out two round areas of enhancement on the left side of the screen.

We nodded.

"I think we can get these with radiation." He paused and stared at the screen, momentarily caught up in his own thoughts, his stance clearly indicating his inner turmoil. He turned back to us. "I don't know how it happened . . ."

Unsure what he was talking about, I was getting worried.

". . . but we missed them. Dr. T and I were both in there, but there was so much . . ." He paused again, and then continued, "I thought we got it all, but somehow we missed those two tumors."

I looked back at the scans. Those two round spots were tumors that remained in Robby's brain. My eyes closed and my head tilted down. When I looked back up, Dr. Solomon was looking regretfully at the scans.

"I . . . I think we can get it with radiation," he repeated, nodding. His voice sounded confident, but his body language didn't convince me. He turned back toward us. "If we have to, we can always go back in again and get them out, but Dr. Cotman is really good at what he does, and I'm sure we can get them with radiation."

I didn't understand why our path had led to this.

"Lord, for two years we have avoided conventional treatment. Why do you want us to do this now?"

Everywhere I'd turned God enforced two words—"Trust Me."

It was out of my hands. There was no other choice. I had to trust.

For six weeks Robby had radiation to his head and spine. Radiating one's head and spine effectively means radiating every vital organ in the body. According to the experts, he was likely to be hospitalized at least once during the course of treatment due to all the side effects. He was certain to have headaches, skin burns, and digestive problems. Resulting weight loss from lack of appetite and mouth sores would threaten his overall health, and his weight was already down to thirty pounds. These were just the definite side effects; many others were possible.

On every visit, outside the outpatient clinic, we would lay hands on him as a family . . . and pray. I clung to the possibility of no side effects. Our church was praying, friends were praying, people across the globe that didn't even know us were praying. In between rounds, Rick would go in and lay hands on Robby and pray as the equipment was repositioned.

Each day we noticed the people around us getting sicker and weaker. Each day they noticed Robby getting stronger and healthier. It was difficult to keep this ambitious six-year-old respectfully still in the waiting area, and even harder to keep him quiet as he ran down the halls to the treatment area, giggling all the way.

He never had a single headache, no stomach problems, and no hospitalizations whatsoever. He never suffered any side effects, save one. The only thing that never occurred to us to pray for was his hair, which eventually diminished—leaving his shiny little scalp in full view. No matter, he was doing well and his hair would eventually grow back.

Once the radiation treatments had ended, Rick and I felt compelled to fast and pray. For seven days we took nothing by mouth except water, still believing for our miracle.

A couple of days later, we went in for Robby's posttreatment appointment. He had another MRI the previous day to determine the effectiveness of the radiation.

"I wanted to show you his scans," said Dr. Cotman, "so we can discuss how to proceed."

He hung up two films side by side for our viewing.

Rick, sitting next to Robby, pointed at the one on the left, "What's that?"

"That is Robby's scan before treatment."

Rick's eyes widened. *"That's* his spine?"

"Yes."

Rick's hand went to his forehead as he bent over in his chair. "I'm going to be sick."

Still standing, I stared at the screen in shock. "We were told there were only a few, small spots . . ."

The image in front of us clearly showed a thick layer of cancer coating Robby's entire spine. My mouth dropped open as I remained motionless, gazing unbelievably at the picture before me.

Rick sat up again and asked, "What is on the right?"

"That's the current scan. We were hoping we could do some spot radiation, but . . ." He sighed, shaking his head before continuing, ". . . there's just too much left."

Rick looked up toward me, his eyes questioning what to do next. I shrugged. We both turned to Dr. Cotman.

"You can still try chemotherapy," he suggested.

"No." I shook my head. "I don't see any point in doing that now. Statistically it doesn't make a difference."

Rick agreed.

Later Rick and I discussed what we should do.

"There's nothing left to do but wait for God to show up and perform a miracle," I said.

"What do you think about the baptism?" he asked.

Our church was having an ocean baptism service that weekend at the beach.

I rolled my eyes. "He's already been baptized."

Rick's eyes filled with skepticism, his head tilted to the side. "I think we should go," he challenged.

"I don't."

"Well, I'm taking him whether you go or not," he warned.

The doctors had cautioned us against placing Robby in water. The port in his chest was now easily seen, as a large hole in his skin had appeared over it. The area itself was red and infected. Water was to be avoided at all costs to prevent sepsis, an infection of the blood that can be fatal. No showers, no baths, and no swimming, they advised.

"You know what the doctors said," I appealed.

"I know, but it doesn't matter anymore. They said they can't do anything else for him, so what difference does it make?"

"I don't think you should do it."

"I do. I can't explain it. I just know it's what God wants us to do."

From that point on, I became angry any time the baptism was mentioned. I still loved and trusted the Lord. I wasn't mad at Him, so it made no sense to me how that topic enraged me, but as the service approached, my attitude toward it worsened. That day came swiftly, and before I knew it we were preparing for an afternoon at the church picnic and baptism.

"Les! Hurry up, we're gonna be late!" Rick called out.

"I'm coming!" I yelled. Anger filled my heart—not even I understood why. I took my sweet time, gradually meeting Rick near the front door. "I don't know why we're going to this stupid thing anyway."

"Are you getting baptized?" he asked teasingly.

I rolled my eyes with disgust. "No," I said bluntly, "I've already been baptized and I don't need to be baptized again."

Smiling, Rick's eyes stared through to my soul as he shook his head.

"Are you getting baptized?" I asked sarcastically.

"Yes, I am," he indicated proudly, "and all the kids are too."

Shaking my head, I took a deep breath and stared at him indignantly. "Whatever."

The ride to the beach was tense. Rick was strong and determined. In spite of his own doubts and fears, he tried to remain upbeat, but my frustrations and anger were set to challenge him. Finally, after all this time, he was confident and bold, certain that this was what God wanted him to do, and I was the one who was a tiny strand from losing all hope.

Arms crossed tightly over my chest, I raged, "I hate the beach!"

"You don't have to go in."

"It's hot and dirty. Sand gets all over everything!"

Rick tried to change the subject. "We're supposed to bring food to share. What do you think we should buy?"

I scowled. "The salt water's all sticky. It makes ya' itch." I paused, then added, "I hate the beach. I've hated it ever since I was little."

"How about fried chicken?"

Rick pulled into the drive-through and ordered a box of chicken. As we waited for our order, my tirade continued. "I'm telling you right now, I'm going stay up in the picnic area. I'm not even going down near that beach. I hate the beach!"

Rick's eyes widened and his authoritarian side took over. "Listen, we're going. That's it! If you don't want to go, you can get out of this van right now!"

Silently I raged inside. I dare not say anything. It was way too far to walk home.

Smiles and hugs were exchanged all afternoon as our church family shared their food, friendship, and love with each other. Picnic tables flourished with the pleasurable sights and smells of a family barbecue. In the background, children squealed with delight in the kiddie pool, older children giggled on the playground, and the young at heart cheered each other on in a game of volleyball. Everyone was having fun.

Admittedly I relished watching Robby play with the other kids, but I wasn't going to let on to Rick that any part of me was enjoying this. For the most part, I was still angry and did not want to be there. The beach lay several football fields away, obscured by the old fort standing on the grounds between the picnic area and the water.

"Hi, Leslie," one of my friends warmly greeted me as I sat alone on the picnic bench. "Are you getting baptized today?"

"Noooo."

Another friend walked up at that moment. "Isn't this awesome?" she oozed.

Yuck! I thought to myself.

"Oh, I *love* these picnics. I can't wait for the baptism. I love the beach!"

"I hate the beach," I flatly responded. Inside I seethed. By now several other friends had gathered around.

"Really?" my friend asked.

"Yes," I answered.

"Why?"

"When I was little, my parents used to spend every weekend at the beach and we'd be there *all* day. They'd pack a picnic lunch and the sandwiches would get soggy and the drinks would get hot and I would get sunburned. I hate the beach."

"I love Pastor Billy's baptism services, don't you?" one friend said to another.

I was not participating in their lovefest. "I don't need to be baptized," I stated matter-of-factly. "I was baptized as a child and I don't see any point in doing it again."

"That's okay," she lovingly reassured me, "you can sit on the beach and watch. You'll love it!"

At 4:00 p.m. the congregation made its way down to the beach.

"You coming?" Rick asked.

Silently I followed along, past the fort and over the boardwalk. Most people were yards ahead. I stopped a few feet onto the sand. The water's edge was easily 100 feet away.

"This is far enough," I informed my family.

Rick helped me lay down a blanket to sit on as the kids took off the clothes they wore over their swimsuits. By this time, Rick's mom had joined us too. Then they all ran happily down to the waves.

I sat by myself, perched on top of a sand dune, far from everyone else. Finally I was beginning to feel some relief. At least now I was alone—just me and my thoughts. With my hat and sunglasses on, my shaded face gave the illusion of my being an invisible observer, far removed from the events on the sandy shore. The sound of the crashing waves and squawking seagulls played into my fallacy as the silent motion picture played in front of me.

Waist deep in the ocean waters, dozens of people, arms raised to the heavens, opened their mouths in praise to the Lord. On the beach, people passed by, unaware of the miraculous occasion about to take place in their presence.

Eventually the mass of people formed a line to our pastor. One by one, they raised their hands to the sky, Pastor would pray, and down they would go.

My anger dissipated as my heart felt joy and appreciation for those who publicly declared their love for Jesus in this beautiful act.

Just as I began to get comfortable, I heard His voice.

"*Get in,*" He said to me.

"Oh, You have got to be kidding me," I answered out loud.

"*Get in.*"

"Are you serious?" I asked aloud.

"*Yes.*"

"*Come on, Lord,*" I pleaded, my mind replaying the preceding conversations of the day. "*I just got done telling everyone how much I hate the beach, and now You want me to get in?*"

"*Yes.*"

I scanned the beach, noticing every single person I would have to walk past to get down there. "*I've already been baptized. Why do I need to do it again?*"

"*You don't have to, but I think you should get in the water.*"

"I'm going to look like such an idiot," I muttered under my breath.

"*Just get in.*"

I had no bathing suit with me and no change of clothes, because I came with no intention of getting anywhere near that water. Having no idea what God wanted or why He wanted me to do this, I only knew that I had to be obedient, no matter how stupid I thought it was or how humiliating it might be.

I stood up on the blanket, hesitating to take the first step. I could only imagine how Rick would react to seeing me down there.

Just do it, I told myself.

Head held high, I marched out to the salty water to join my family in line. When I approached, Rick was facing the other direction. His mom smiled but said nothing.

"Mommy!" Robby called out.

Rick turned around and smiled, staring at me for a moment, smirking—his mind obviously assessing the situation. I knew he was going to make some smart-alecky comment.

Instead he nodded and turned back around, but after several minutes in the extensive line, he could no longer contain his wonder. "Why did you get in?" he asked me.

"I'll tell you later."

"Are you getting baptized?"

I shrugged my shoulders and smiled.

Time quickly passed and eventually I watched as one at a time my mother-in-law, my children, and then my husband were each baptized.

Then Pastor Billy turned to me. "Are you getting baptized today?"

I nodded.

An avid swimmer since the age of six, I wasn't afraid of the water; I *loved* swimming. Yet my heart raced as I nervously awaited my turn under the water's surface.

"Do you know Jesus?" Pastor Billy asked me.

"Yes."

"Does He live in your heart?"

I nodded.

"What's He mean to you?"

"Everything," I replied.

My mind wandered as I began recalling Pastor's jokes about holding people under. Distracted by my own thoughts, I barely heard him say to me, "When you go under I want you to count to three, okay?"

I nodded.

"And when you do that, I want you to release everything. Just let it all go and leave it down at the bottom of the sea. Alright?"

I had no idea what he was talking about, but nodded in agreement anyway.

"Raise your hands," he told me.

With my hands in the air and my eyes closed, my nervousness increased. I couldn't wait to get this over with.

Then Pastor began to pray, "Holy Ghost, we thank You. We praise You. We give You glory. Master, we thank You today for

Leslie, and we ask, Jesus, that You would let all the pain and the guilt of the past be gone away. Wash and clean her. Set her free and make her a new woman. We baptize you in the name of the Father, in the name of the Son, and in the name of the Holy Ghost."

Gently he dunked me under the water.

I counted. One . . . two . . . three.

Bam!

My limp body was raised from the water by deacons and elders.

"Something broke! Something broke, Rick!" I heard the pastor yell.

The power of God hit me so hard that I don't even remember being carried from the water. The next thing I knew, I was lying on the beach. Wet sand was in my hair and broken shells clung to my salt-covered skin. An elder's wife lovingly prayed for me as I wept. Eventually she covered me with a towel and then left to tend to someone else. I don't know how long I lay there, but when I finally got up, Rick was standing over me, smiling.

"Are you okay?" he asked.

I wasn't sure what to say or how to answer. My body tingled and my insides felt like they were floating in a liquid pool of love. I'd never felt this way before. As the sensations overcame me, my mind struggled for the right words. The only thing that made it to my lips was a breathy, "Wow!"

I didn't yet realize it, but I had emerged from the watery cocoon transformed. Whatever ugliness accompanied me that day, it now laid buried deep on the ocean floor, carried away by a mighty wave of living water.

15
THE WORD

High upon a hill, in the most beautiful land ever seen, sat the palace of the king. The illustrious, colossal building was arrayed in splendor—the most glorious structure in all the land. Inside, preparations were underway for the magnificent ceremony, marking the end of a long and difficult apprenticeship.

The king's court overflowed with countless noble peers set to witness the one who would be admitted to the chivalric elite. Within the great hall, the sun's rays shined through picturesque stained-glass windows, brightly glimmering off the golden fixtures and many jewels that graced the palatial expanse.

Trumpets blared, declaring the entrance of his majesty, and all who heard bowed down before him. He entered with nobility and grace, the epitome of gallantry. Adorned in the finest linens, a well-trimmed beard, and perfect manicure, his highness sat down gracefully upon his royal throne.

Moments later, the halls filled with the sound of a sword clanking in unison with footsteps; before long the summoned squire entered. Having lived a life dedicated to truth, honor, courage, generosity, and humility, this person was about to receive the highest commendation. Approaching the throne, this one for whom the celebratory event had been held bowed down before the king.

"My Lord."

The king rose from his throne to address his loyal subject. As the king looked upon this one, recounting the depths from which this prodigal had come, unbound love and appreciation poured from his eyes.

"This world is overwrought with the effects of darkness, but you have been set apart and have lived a life in opposition to these powerful forces," the king declared. With head bowed and eyes closed, the squire relished in the moment, grateful to be counted worthy of the king's honor and affection. Taking his sword in hand, the king tapped the squire once upon each shoulder, knowing his beloved child had given all toward a job well done. "Arise, my faithful servant. This day you shall see your reward."

Leaving the beach, we delighted in the fantastic experience of our day. Still reveling in the warmth of God's embrace, an intense love continued to surround me. I turned from my seat in the front of the van to look back upon Robby's sun-kissed face. An uncontrollable smile took over my lips while I admired the glow that radiated from him. In that moment, nothing else mattered. We were a happy family—whether together on this earth or temporarily separated by space and time. Our love was strong enough to bridge any divide.

My eyes scanned over my son's body, intently taking in the happiness he exuded. As my glance fell to his chest, I stared lovingly at the spot in his skin where his port was. A new layer of skin now covered the hole through which the port was easily seen only hours ago.

"I can't believe that hole is gone," I remarked to Rick.

"Is the skin still there?" Rick asked for reassurance.

With a wink and a smile sent in Robby's direction, I answered, "Sure is!"

I noticed the change in Robby's skin a short time after the baptism, while Rick and I watched Robby splashing and playing blissfully on the beach. His tiny squeals and giggles filled the air, mimicking the sounds of elation echoing joyously in my heart. No more hole, no redness, no swelling, and no pus—nothing! Only a small, pink spot of new skin remained in its place. We were in awe, regularly double-checking to reaffirm what our eyes were seeing.

Defying all medical prognoses, Robby continued getting stronger during the weeks following that amazing day. Increasingly, he was returning to the energetic, happy child we knew before this nightmare ever began. Part of me believed that the war was finally over; something inside me was certain that the hole in Robby's skin wasn't the only thing to disappear that day. Still, another part of me was afraid to trust it. How many times over the past two years had I believed for the best, only to find out the cancer was back?

Up until that time, I had only lost two people in my life that I was close to. One was a special woman who babysat me when I was young. She often said that she fell in love with me while I was still a baby. Over time she became a second mother to me. Her passing saddened me for many years. The other loss was my grandmother, who died when I was pregnant with Robby. Both their deaths resulted from cancer. They had different types, but each died soon after the cancer affected their spines. Those memories anguished me from the time I first learned that Robby's cancer had spread to his spine too.

I did my best to squelch those tormenting thoughts with all I'd learned from scripture over the past two years. I forgave everyone who'd ever wronged me and, in turn, repented and asked the Lord to forgive me of my sins. Nightly family prayer, combined with daily praise and worship, was now a routine part of our lives.

One of Grandma's hand-crocheted handkerchiefs, with her name, Mary, embroidered across the corner, was given to Pastor Billy to wear during a healing service weeks earlier. Robby slept with the anointing-soaked cloth on his pillow every night.

For the last six months, I too had my own private ritual, going before the Lord each night in prayer to practice giving testimony of Robby's healing—a testimony I planned to share one day with everyone I could. Anything we were aware of that we were supposed to do, we did. We had done our part. Now all that was left was for us to trust and wait for God to do His.

Six weeks passed, and Robby was in the MRI machine once again. By this time we had grown confident that Robby was healed, but I was reluctant to put my whole heart into it. I had to have proof. I needed so badly to see that the tumors had disappeared from the scans—I longed to hear the doctor say all was well.

The next day, we went to Dr. Solomon's office for the results. He was smiling and happy as he walked into the room. "Whatever you're doing, keep doing it!" he encouraged. "The scans are clean."

Rick and I smiled knowingly at each other. There were no fireworks, and the doctor did not pronounce Robby forever healed, but reality doesn't often follow the outline of a movie script. Life is filled with uncertainty, and the only way to be sure of anything is to follow God's great plan for each of us.

In our hearts we knew that Robby was finally healed. Hand in hand our entire family raced to the elevator, laughing and giggling all the way. The war was finally over.

With our bags packed, we left that weekend for our long-overdue vacation—more than ready for an extended celebration.

Weeks later . . . I had returned to working part-time in the evenings. One night when I got home, Rick was waiting up for me.

"You're not going to believe this," Rick said.

"What?" I asked.

"Come sit down with me," Rick urged.

I grabbed a cold glass of water and sat with him at the dining room table. "So, what is it?"

"When I got home this evening, I was sitting here talking with my mom," he started.

"Yeah?"

"Robby was sitting on her lap playing with his transformer, and Mom was telling me a story about someone she knew who saw an angel."

"Cool."

"Oh, wait 'til you hear this," he enthused. "Anyhow, we're sitting here talking, and Robby's just sitting there playing with his little toy, when all of a sudden he said, 'I've seen Jesus.'"

"Really?" I asked while questioning Rick with my eyes, wondering if he was making this up. "When?"

"Well, Mom and I looked at each other with our eyes wide with surprise, and we motioned to each other not to break his concentration on his toy because we wanted to find out what he was talking about."

"Yes."

Rick continued, "And I said, 'You did?' and Robby said, 'Yes.' And then I asked, 'When did you see him?' and he answered, 'At my last operation.' "

"Are you serious?" I asked.

"Yes! I wanted to question him—I didn't want him to know I was quizzing him, but I had to know the truth."

"Okay . . ."

"So then I said, 'Well, what did He look like?' and he said, 'He was shiny.' "

"Shiny?"

"Yeah, shiny. I guess that was the best way he could describe what he saw."

"Makes sense."

"And I said, 'What do you mean—shiny?' He shrugged and said, 'He shined.' "

"Wow."

"The whole time he's still playing with his toy and talking very matter-of-fact, like it was no big deal."

"So did he say anything else?"

"Yeah. So then I asked, 'What was He wearing?' and he said, 'A white bathrobe.' "

"A white bathrobe?" I laughed.

"Well, you know . . . that's probably what it looked like to him."

"Yeah," I nodded in agreement.

"Then I asked, 'What did He have on His feet?' and he said, 'Sandals.' So I asked, 'What color were they?' and he said, 'They were shiny—like metal.' "

"What was your mom doing all this time?" I asked.

"She was just sitting there smiling, listening to the whole thing. Ya' know . . . I was trying to shoot holes in his story. I figured he wouldn't have the answers."

"Why?"

"He's only six. And I figured he'd get to the point that he'd give up and say, 'I don't know.' But he never did—he knew!!"

I smiled as I continued to listen.

Rick went on. "Then I asked him, 'What did his hair look like?' "

" 'It was long,' "

" 'What color was it?' "

" 'It shined.' "

"Then I asked him, 'What was He doing?' Robby said, 'Holding me.' "

My eyes widened in amazement. "Holding him?" I echoed.

Rick nodded and continued with his story. "So I said, 'Well, what were you doing?' and he said, 'I was sitting on his lap.' I asked, 'Which leg?' and he said, 'This one.' " Rick pointed to his right leg. "Then I asked him, 'Where were Jesus' arms?' and Robby said, 'His arm was holding me.' Finally I asked, 'Was anyone else there?' and he said, 'No . . . but there was music.' "

"Wow . . . how cool is that?"

"I know, right? This whole time he's just sitting there playing with his toy. He never even looked up. So I asked him, 'Then what happened?' Robby answered, 'He told me it was time to go back with Mommy and Daddy.' "

I was in awe. I smiled as I thought, *Robby sat on Jesus' lap. Wow!*

Rick finished, "My mom and I looked at each other in amazement. We didn't say much because we didn't want to ruin the moment. Then Robby slid off her lap and went off playing."

"That is amazing!"

"Yes, I know. Then I remembered when Robby was going into his last surgery and we prayed that Jesus would protect him and keep him safe."

"Looks like the answer was yes." I smiled.

Indeed it was. Although we believed Robby was healed, only the passing of time with no recurrence would ever really prove our belief to be true.

It's now been thirteen years since Robby's healing. The cancer is gone and has never returned—hallelujah!!

Before any of this ever happened, I lived a pretty average life by most people's standards. I grew up in a middle-class home, went to public school, and did all the usual things middle-class people do.

Our Christianity was mediocre as well. We knew about Jesus, but didn't spend much time with Him. Like many, we had Him over for Christmas and Easter, and were sure to call whenever we had a crisis, but we didn't really need Him around for much else.

My parents divorced when I was twelve, and growing into maturity in a single-parent home was a challenge. As the oldest of three children, I was the one positioned for a large share of responsibility. Though it may have been good for me in many respects, the weight of it became overwhelming, and eventually I became resentful and rebellious. In time I became jaded by the disappointments of life and hardened by a bigger dissatisfaction with people. I had grown to believe that, for the most part, the world was a horrible place filled with mean, selfish people who didn't care about anyone but themselves.

Don't get me wrong. I didn't spend all of my waking hours angry with the world. I accepted that this was just the way the world was. My own small circle of friends and family shared life's joys with me—that was all I needed.

Then I got deathly ill and suddenly I needed God again. I begged and pleaded for mercy. I wanted to be well. My baby needed me, my boys needed me, and my husband needed me. I promised God that if He healed me, I would be good and would eat right and take care of my body. I promised Him that I wouldn't forget about Him and would do whatever He wanted.

Eventually the doctors performed exploratory surgery to discover that the object inside of me was an abdominal abscess, one liter in size. It filled my gut, shutting down my digestive tract, nearly killing me. Where it came from or why, the doctors could never figure out. Once removed, I quickly regained my health, returning home days later, though it would take several months for me to regain the strength to become my former self. Before long, I was back to my old ways, absorbed in the details of my day-to-day living.

Then Robby got sick and I found myself with needs far beyond anything I could've ever imagined or predicted. To my amazement, numerous people stepped up to bless our lives and lend a helping hand.

At events, children showered Robby with gifts of clothes, toys, and other treasures from their heart. One little boy, about twelve years old, approached me at one of these events and told me he was praying for Robby to be healed. A gold chain with a large pendant of an eagle hung around his neck. He removed it and handed it to me.

"I want Robby to have this," he told me.

"Oh honey, thank you. But don't you want to keep this?" I asked.

He didn't look like his family had much of their own, and I felt guilty taking this little boy's treasure. But he was resolute in his request, and the look in his eyes let me know that I would cause him more pain by refusing his generosity than by accepting it.

Another time, a young sailor on leave came to a fund-raising event. On bended knee he proudly showed Robby the two pins he had worked hard to be awarded. "I'm just a poor sailor. I don't have much, but I want to give you something," he said, handing Robby his sailor cap with both pins firmly attached. It was the young man's most prized possession.

"Here, Robby, I want you to have this," he insisted. "Promise me you'll wear it."

Robby nodded, smiling ear to ear.

"When you do, remember how strong you are."

The agony of those two years was comforted by the regular, heartfelt generosity of others. Many, many people played a part in our miracle. And even though we didn't always see eye to eye with some of the doctors, we know they too did their very best to help Robby the only way they knew how.

Though at one point in time I thought humankind was the pits—that is no longer the case. I believe, and I want you to know, that there are good people in the world, people who care about you and what you are going through, and they want to help you too.

Whatever you may be struggling with in your life, be assured that God has individuals lined up to help you along the way. His divine plan may contain a multitude or maybe only a few. Whatever He decides, be open to it. Don't discount the power and ability that God can place into even a single person. You don't need hundreds or even dozens of people to overcome and achieve success. One person with passion can change the world.

Along my journey, I have learned the value of the power one person can have in affecting the lives of others, and I'm reminded how this has proven true all along our country's amazing history. Repeatedly, throughout recorded times, the decisions of one individual changed the destiny of countless others:

- One man dared to brave the vast ocean, discovering the New World.
- One president dared to stand for equality, bringing true freedom to America and *all* her citizens.
- One inventor with a passion made electric light available to every home around the world.

In our story, many "ones" made an impact on our destiny too:

- One man had the foresight to see we would need money beyond our own means.
- One doctor fought for decades to make available a nontoxic cancer treatment for those desiring an alternative to traditional cancer therapies.
- One pastor, an example of the healing power of Jesus, gave us hope and inspiration and encouraged us to stand in faith.

For all of us there are even more important Ones:

- One Father who gave His Son, a ransom for many.
- One Savior who sacrificed His life so that we could live with Him forever.
- One Holy Spirit who guides our lives from glory to glory.

Like me, you too can be one person whose decision today will affect a multitude tomorrow. Some would say that I was an inherently strong person. I had just survived a health crisis of my own, had three kids (one of whom was a new baby), worked a full-time job—and suddenly a child with cancer.

I can only say that I don't deserve credit for superhuman strength. I look back on parts of this story with the same level of bewilderment as you, for I wasn't driven by logic. What I had was not some natural talent, innate specialness, or advanced training. It was a power beyond my own human strength, sourced by an inner wisdom that rose up within me.

There's nothing special about me. As you've read, I'm not flawless. I smoked and cussed—and I wish those were the worst things I'd ever done. I've had times when my faith wavered, when fear prevailed. At times I was downright angry with God. I am an ordinary person just like you, yet the same strength that rose within me is available to you too.

You see, I tried to be tough, but in the end I found out I wasn't strong enough. I couldn't be good enough or love enough. I would never be smart enough. No matter what I tried, my success was dependent on the Lord, for His strength is made perfect in our weakness.[1]

Many of us wonder why some people do not survive such trials, as Robby did. Perhaps they found it difficult to believe in God's desire to heal them. Maybe they ignored His signals regarding the correct path to take. Or possibly, it simply was their appointed time, having fulfilled all they were called to do on the earth.

The truth is: I don't know. I don't have all the answers, but I know the One who does. By far, the single best decision I made was to turn to Jesus—the strength that lives on the inside of me. With Him, even my mistakes could be made into something good.

Growing up I learned the Apostles' Creed, a profession of faith that includes the belief that Jesus will come again in glory to judge the living and the dead. As I travelled the road of this journey, I often pictured myself standing in front of Jesus, in all His glory and majesty, on the Day of Judgment. When those around me told me to be realistic, I wondered what I would say to Jesus on that day. When I felt like doctors were trying to manipulate and guilt trip me into decisions, I saw myself kneeling before His throne and imagined what it would be like. How would I answer to Him? I knew the day would come when I would be held accountable for each decision I was making. Would I be explaining how difficult it was for me to make decisions in the face of adversity? That I allowed the spirit of fear to rule over me rather than the Spirit of the living God? Or would He say to me that which my heart longed to hear: "Well done, thou good and faithful servant!"[2]? Seeing these images in my mind's eye gave me courage to stand up for what I knew was right, even when seemingly everyone around me was convinced I was wrong. I had to follow my king, for I would ultimately answer to Him alone.

He brightly lit our path, giving us access to many resources we otherwise wouldn't have achieved on our own. But the steps that we took are not a cure-all for terminal illness. Natural interventions that worked for us will not necessarily work for you or your loved ones. Though many of the methodologies we employed are both useful and widely accepted, there is no magic bullet in nature or medicine. The real key is to find the Lord's path for you.

"In 2007, 11 million people worldwide were diagnosed with cancer and nearly 8 million people died from cancer."[3] While advances in medicine have improved five-year survival rates, long-term survival rates remain dismal. Both the incidence and death rates from cancer are expected to increase in coming years—yet there is hope. Although doctors, medicines, vitamins, and the like are useful, they are but tools of the Master. Doctors can operate and medicate, but there's a reason they cannot guarantee success: only Jesus has the power to *heal.* No matter what war you are fighting to survive right now, He is able to help you like no other. One day you will appear before His throne, and when you do, He's not going to ask you how big your house was or how much money you made. He won't ask you how many friends you had or how many good deeds you did. He won't even ask what church you went to. He knows all about you. The question is: Do you know Him?

He longs for a moment-by-moment relationship with you—a special bond where you share every detail of your day, one where you learn to put your life trustfully in His hands. He wants to give you victory in the big things—and the little ones too.

Though this book is ending, your story is just beginning. Wherever you are, whatever you've done, Jesus loves you—you don't have to struggle through your days alone. He has great plans for you! Let Him write the pages of your life; He can change your story. He believes in you and His love for you is never ending.

Don't wait another minute to seek Him. Decide to follow—wherever He may lead. Ask Him to illuminate your path. Then whatever He tells you to do—do it![4] And soon *your* story will be impacting the lives of others too.

Don't ever give up, no matter what. Press on! So that when the appointed time arrives, you'll bow down before the King of kings—and on bended knee, to account for all that you've become—you'll be one to hear "Well done!"

AFTERWORD

I'll tell you something about cancer. Once it's been in your body, it has an effect on you like nothing else. You experience it all: fear, loneliness, anger . . . all of it. And if you're a parent of a child with cancer, the whole family is greatly impacted.

This remarkable story of Robby Graham and his healing miracle—a story of faith in God, prayer, and divine intervention—reminds all of us to reach beyond the limitations of human resources.

You too can have access to this supernatural connection with God, the same as Robby did. Today ask Jesus Christ to come into your heart and forgive the past. Allow Him to be the navigating force for your life. As Robby and his family found out, so will you, that Jesus has the power and **He is faithful** to see you through *any* challenge.

Billy Burke
Senior Pastor
Miracle Center World Outreach
Tampa, FL

ACKNOWLEDGEMENTS

All those who supported us during this trying time deserve to be honored for their generous efforts. Too numerous to name individually, I'd like to at least acknowledge some bighearted works not yet mentioned in this story.

I remember the first time we brought Robby home. Midway Plumbing (Clearwater, Florida) generously provided the equipment and labor needed to remodel our dilapidated bathroom, free of charge, so he could bathe in a safe environment.

Then the fund-raisers began. It is difficult to convey the enormity of appreciation we have for the multitude of people who donated money, many anonymously. There were those who coordinated fund-raisers and those who donated to the events—golf tournaments, firefighter nights at the local wing house, antique car shows, and a bowl-a-thon, to name a few. Individuals and celebrities alike contributed to a hugely successful dinner-dance and auction as well.

The entertainers at some of these events—in particular, support from Mason Dixon, Nancy Alexander, and 100.7 KISSFM radio, along with reporters of various news organizations—helped spread the word about our plight and extended our reach far beyond our own sphere of influence.

Our love and good wishes are gratefully extended to Jill Marie and the drivers and crews of Sunshine Speedway who were

169

generous supporters and fans of Robby. Even stock cars carried Robby Graham's name and fund-raising information.

We also received an outpouring of love, prayers, and fundraising efforts from: Faith Academy (Robby's preschool) as well as St. Patrick's Catholic School and Church, and our friends and family at the Miracle Center Church.

Words cannot express our immense appreciation for Christians of all denominations who cried out in prayer on our behalf. Countless times people cooked us food and babysat our children. Offers to paint our house, buy new tires for our van, and the like came in regularly. December 1997, unbeknownst to even those closest to us, was particularly tight financially. Miraculously, the Seminole Fire Department felt led to step in, providing an abundance of food and toys for our family that Christmas.

I don't know that we can ever truly convey the gratitude we have for key players in our story, but I'd like to at least attempt to honor them again here:

- Mike Silver, our knight in shining armor. God has great plans for you! Thank you also to your precious family: Bonnie, Heather and Kimmie. You were all there for us when we needed you. We don't know what we would've done without you.

- Lealman Fire District, Pinellas Park Fire Department, Pinellas Suncoast Fire District and all the firefighters and Sheriff deputies (and your wives) who worked fund-raisers and more. Thank you for your hard work and sacrifice. We appreciate you more than words can say.

- Dr. Solomon, the best neurosurgeon ever, thank you for your dedication and for being there when we needed you most.

- Dr. Burzynski, for paying the price. We continue to pray for you and your patients.

- Dr. Friedman, a great man and a great doctor who continues to devote his life to finding a cure for cancer.

- Mom, for all the encouragement and happy thoughts. Thanks, Mom!

- To my sister Candy and sister-in-law Christine, thank you for all the help, late nights on the telephone, and more. Your support kept me sane.
- Dad, for coming through when it counted. Your actions changed our lives. Thank you, Daddy!
- Pastor Billy, you're the single greatest example (besides Jesus) of how to live a holy life. Thank you for your faith, your prayers, and your love.
- Rick's mom, Sharron, you are an amazing woman. Thank you for all you did to enrich our lives. We miss you!

For those who made the telling of this story a reality, may God bless each of you beyond your wildest dreams! Janis Whipple, my amazing editor; Wanda Downey, who edited through the painful early versions; Lisa Broesh, Karri Head, Lois Knetchges, Michelle Brody, and Kent Smith for reading and giving your heartfelt input.

To my amazing children: Ricky, you helped your brother more than you'll ever know. Amanda, you're the best baby girl ever. Robby, you inspire me to greatness. I'm still in awe of your remarkable strength. Andrew, your healing is next! I love you all.

To my wonderful husband: I thank the Lord for you every day. I couldn't have done any of this without you and can't wait to see what more God has for me to do with you.

A very special thank you to my great friend Shelly Ballestero for your encouragement, input and connections. You are such a blessing!

And most importantly, to Jesus, for paying the ultimate price. May I always stay mindful of Your love and commitment. Help me to share You with the world. They need You now more than ever.

END NOTES

Chapter 6

1. "One Sweet Day," written by Mariah Carey, Walter Afanasieff, Wanya Morris, Shawn Stockman, Nathan Morris, and Michael McCary, performed and recorded by Mariah Carey and Boyz II Men, *Daydream*, 1995, Columbia Records.

2. "I Will Remember You," written by Sarah McLachlan, Séamus Egan, and Dave Merenda, performed and recorded by Sarah McLachlan, soundtrack to *The Brothers McMullen*, 1995, Fox Searchlight.

3. Julian Whitaker, "Everyone's Health Is at Stake If We Lose This Therapy," *Health and Healing Newsletter*, suppl. (mid-February), 1, 4.

4. Ibid.

5. Ibid.

6. Ibid.

7. Ibid.

8. Ibid.

9. *Lorenzo's Oil*, directed by George Miller (Hollywood, CA: Universal Studios, 1992).

10. J. Balter-Seri, C. Mor, A. Shuper, R. Zaizov, and I. J. Cohen, "Cure of recurrent medulloblastoma: the contribution of surgical resection at relapse," *PubMed.gov*, March 15, 1997, http://www.ncbi.nlm.nih.gov/pubmed/9070504?ordinalpos=14&it ool=
EntrezSystem2.PEntrez.Pubmed.Pubmed_ResultsPanel.Pubmed_D efaultReportPanel
.Pubmed_RVDDocSum (accessed August 19, 2010).

Chapter 7

1. Information for this section taken from: *Encyclopedia Britannica Online*, s.v. "Titanic," http://Britannica.com/titanic/01–01.html (accessed August 19, 2010); "The Titanic Construction," *Titanic-Facts.com*, http://wwwtitanic-facts.com/titanic-construction.html (accessed August 19, 2010); and "Titanic's Watertight Compartments," *Titanic-Titanic.com*, http://www.titanic-titanic.com/titanic_watertight_compartments
.shtml (accessed August 19, 2010).

Chapter 9

1. JoAnn Levy, "The Elephant," http://www.goldrush.com/~joann/elephant.htm, (accessed August 19, 2010).

2. "Seeing the Elephant," Nantucket Historical Association, http://www.nha.org/history/hn/HNelephant.htm (accessed August 19, 2010).

3. Levy, "The Elephant."

Chapter 11

1. Witham, Larry, "Cancer Doctor Sees Pope, but Not about His Health," *The Washington Times*, September 26, 1996, A12.

2. Congressman Peter DeFazio, personal letter, January 3, 1997.

3. Charles, Zewe, "Cancer Doctor on Trial in Houston," CNN Interactive, http://cnn.com/HEALTH/9701/07/nfm/cancer.doc/index.html#2 (accessed August 19, 2010).

Chapter 12

1. *Apollo 13*, VHS, directed by Ron Howard (Hollywood, CA: Universal Studios, 1995).

2. Philippians 4:8, KJV.

3. *Apollo 13*.

Chapter 13

1. Information for this section taken from: Gerald Beals, "The Biography of Thomas Edison, 1999, *ThomasEdison.com*, http://thomasedison.com/biography.html (accessed August 19, 2010); *Wikipedia*, s.v. "Milan, Ohio," http://en.wikipedia.org/wiki/Milan, Ohio *(accessed August 19, 2010); Ker Than,* "How the Human Eye Works," November 28, 2005, *LiveScience.com*, Health section, http://www.livescience.com/health/051128eye_works.html (accessed August 19, 2010); and Craig Freudenrich, PhD, "How Light Works," *HowStuffWorks.com*, A Discovery Company, http://science.howstuffworks.com/light.htm (accessed August 19, 2010).

Chapter 14

1. *Wizard of Oz*, directed by Victor Fleming (Culver City, CA: MGM Studios, 1939).

Chapter 15

1. See 2 Corinthians 12:9, KJV.

2. Matthew 25:23, KJV.

3. *Policy and Action for Cancer Prevention, Food, Nutrition, and Physical Activity: A Global Perspective* (Washington, DC: World Cancer Research Fund/American Institute for Cancer Research, 2009), 4.

4. See John 2:5, KJV.

ABOUT THE AUTHOR

Leslie Graham is a devoted mother of four and happily married wife of twenty-three years. Her life today is the American dream, but she has had more than her fair share of tragedy and crisis. Having suffered losses in both her career and personal life, she knows the pain and challenges that many face. Against all odds, she and her husband joined forces to cross the barriers from poverty to prosperity. This journey included the monumental task of helping their four-year-old son battle and defeat "terminal" brain cancer. In the process of this incredible journey, divine intervention changed her life forever, transforming her into a true giver whose caring nature and relentless passion now drive her as a champion for the afflicted.

This ambassador of love, whose heart beats as a humble servant seeking to help others, persistently travels the country conducting workshops and seminars to support and spread the messages contained in Beyond Boo-Boo Kisses.

Leslie's compassion for others, years of wisdom and experience, and enthusiastic, fun-loving personality, combined with her love and reverence for God, is the fuel that pushes her to help others reach the highest heights.

We invite you to learn more about Leslie and view photos related to this story by visiting her website: **www.momsmentor.com**.

You want to make a difference
We want to help!

Make a Difference . . .

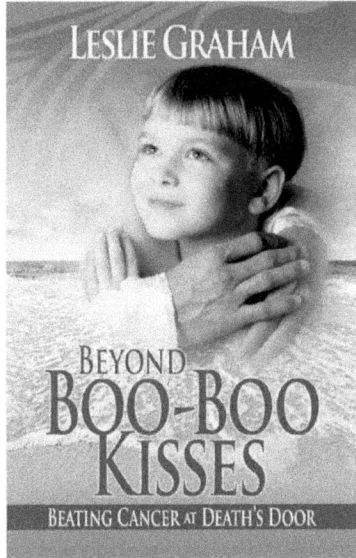

. . . where your heart is

We're Sharing 50% of the profits!!

Share the miracle AND Create a significant income for your favorite organization.

Call Now to Learn How!
The Robby Graham Foundation
1-800-743-0363
RGF@momsmentor.com

www.ingramcontent.com/pod-product-compliance
Lightning Source LLC
Chambersburg PA
CBHW050120280326
41933CB00010B/1181